HEAL YOUR
— ORAL —
MICROBIOME

T0307085

HEAL YOUR
—ORAL—
MICROBIOME

Balance and Repair Your Mouth Microbes to
Improve Gut Health, Reduce Inflammation and Fight Disease

— CASS NELSON-DOOLEY, M.S. —

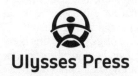

Ulysses Press

Text copyright © 2019 Cass Nelson-Dooley. Design and concept copyright © 2019 Ulysses Press and its licensors. All rights reserved. Any unauthorized duplication in whole or in part or dissemination of this edition by any means (including but not limited to photocopying, electronic devices, digital versions, and the internet) will be prosecuted to the fullest extent of the law.

Published in the United States by:
Ulysses Press
P.O. Box 3440
Berkeley, CA 94703
www.ulyssespress.com

ISBN: 978-1-61243-900-6
Library of Congress Catalog Number: 2018967977

Printed in Canada by Marquis Book Printing
10 9 8 7 6 5 4 3 2 1

Acquisitions editor: Bridget Thoreson
Managing editor: Claire Chun
Project editor: Renee Rutledge
Copyeditor: Shayna Keyles
Proofreader: Lauren Harrison
Indexer: Sayre Van Young
Front cover design: Malea Clark-Nicholson
Interior design: what!design @ whatweb.com
Interior art: page 52 © Jake Nelson-Dooley. Remaining artwork from
    shutterstock.com—page 29 © Iconic Bestiary; pages 31, 69
    © ilusmedical; pages 65, 91 © Blamb; page 72 © Sergii
    Kuchugurnyi; pages 77, 110 © Elen Bushe; page 103 © alphabe
    (mouth), © Alila Medical Media (head)
Production: Jake Flaherty

Distributed by Publishers Group West

IMPORTANT NOTE TO READERS: This book has been written and published for informational and educational purposes only. It is not intended to serve as medical advice or to be any form of medical treatment. You should always consult with your physician before altering or changing any aspect of your medical treatment. Do not stop or change any prescription medications without the guidance and advice of your physician. Any use of the information in this book is made on the reader's good judgment and is the reader's sole responsibility. This book is not intended to diagnose or treat any medical condition and is not a substitute for a physician. This book is independently authored and published and no sponsorship or endorsement of this book by, and no affiliation with, any trademarked brands or other products mentioned within is claimed or suggested. All trademarks that appear in ingredient lists and elsewhere in this book belong to their respective owners and are used here for informational purposes only. The author and publisher encourage readers to patronize the quality brands mentioned in this book.

CONTENTS

THE CONVERGENCE OF THE MICROBIOME, NATURE, AND HEALTH

I trace the origins of this book all the way back to my grand-parents' farm in northern Louisiana. My grandmother baked pie from blueberries we picked by hand in the yard. My grandfather prided himself on his vegetable gardens. He and I discussed organic gardening and how you could work with nature, not against it, to get healthier food. The dark, rich soil full of microbes, the insects, the plants, the sun, and the rain all seemed to work together in perfect harmony.

Not long into my premedical tract at the University of Georgia, I found myself drawn to natural treatments for disease. I was fascinated to learn that over 75 percent of our modern-day pharmaceuticals originally came from plants, animals, or microorganisms. Nature offers treatments to our most terrifying ailments, including cancer.

Intrigued, I set about studying medicinal plants with the hopes of preserving cultural knowledge, conserving ecosystems, and finding new treatments for disease. I earned my master of science in ethnopharmacology researching ancient rainforest remedies in the jungles of Panama with medicine men and women. I worked in laboratories trying to find the next new pharmaceutical drug from nature.

My background in plant medicine and pharmacy (and a friendship with the owners' daughter) led me to Metametrix Clinical Laboratory, where I consulted with physicians about their patients' laboratory tests. These cutting-edge assessments could tell if a person had healthy levels of vitamins, minerals, and hormones; whether they had food sensitivities; or if their gut microbiome was out of balance. With these tests we could identify root causes of disease that, once corrected, could change lives forever.

We were no longer bound to "prescription pad medicine," as world-renown integrative and functional medicine leader Dr. Sidney Baker calls it. This seeks primarily to label a disease with a diagnosis and treat the symptoms with a prescription. Instead, we were looking for and fixing the underlying causes of disease. I met physicians who were curing the incurable. They looked for systems in the body that were broken, removed the bad stuff, replaced the good stuff, and turned around serious health conditions.

I wasn't the only one interested in a better kind of medicine. There was a movement happening in our country that is still happening to this day. People want better health and they want it without side effects. They don't want to take a handful of prescription medications every day. Evidence of this movement is in the nutritional supplement industry. Driven solely by consumer demand, this industry was worth at least $6 billion in 1996 and has grown to over $18 billion. Power to the people.

The fuel for this movement is knowledge.

I like to think that the information in this book contributes in a small way to the growing demand for better health alternatives across the globe. This book will help you understand and address the microbiome, which can be a major underlying cause of illness. As you read this book you will get answers, understanding, action steps, a lot of scientific evidence, and, hopefully, a little entertainment. I want to ignite your wonder about the magnificent microbiome and give you treatment ideas to restore your microbial health without unwanted side effects.

It's an exciting time for knowledge, technology, and a new standard for optimum wellness. Thank you for picking up this book and taking a deeper look.

CHAPTER 1

THE MAGNIFICENT MICROBIOME

*"If you don't like bacteria,
you're on the wrong planet."*
—Stewart Brand, American photographer and writer

Inside your mouth are millions and millions of tiny bugs. Most of them are harmless, many of them are very beneficial, and a few of them cause diseases. Imagine your mouth, teeming with these invisible bugs. If this gives you the willies, you aren't the only one. We have a long history of hating bacteria and seeing them as the bad guys that cause infections, fever, pain, and suffering. But we have learned in recent decades that many of these bacteria are *good for* us.

The truth is, we are not just human beings. We are super-organisms. According to "The Oral Microbiome—An Update for Oral Healthcare Professionals," "for millions of years, our resident microbes have coevolved and coexisted with us in a mostly harmonious symbiotic relationship. We are not distinct entities from our microbiome, but together we form a 'superorganism'... with the microbiome playing a significant role in our physiology and health." We carry around trillions of microscopic bugs all day, every day, for our whole lives. These microbes help us fight disease, boost our nutrition, protect us from infections, and tune the metabolism.

It turns out that there are about as many bacterial cells in the body as there are human cells, though many scientists believe the number of bacterial cells may be even higher. There are millions of bacteria in every crack and crevice of the body. They inhabit most organs of the body, especially the ones that are open to the outside world, like the gastrointestinal tract, skin, eyes, genitals, and more.

"Microbiome," "Microbiota," or "Bugs?"

The bacteria, viruses, fungi, and other microscopic organisms that live inside and on your body make up your *microbiota*. The DNA codes (or genomes) of those bugs make up your *microbiome*.[1] However, when we are talking about a community of bugs that lives inside the body, we also call it a microbiome. You'll see this word over and over again, so it's worth remembering. The human microbiome is a super-hot area of research. It's like exploring a whole new universe—one that lives within.

I often use the word "microbiome" to talk about the microbes or microscopic organisms that live all over and inside of you. But sometimes I think it's simpler to just call them "bugs." Don't let that word—bugs—scare you off. The majority of your microbiome is made up of good bugs. And we aren't talking about insects.

THE MICROBIOME BREAKDOWN

When we talk about the human microbiome, bacteria are the major players. Bacteria are single-cell organisms that don't have the same cellular makeup that we do. Bacteria are tiny. If you line up 1,000 bacterial cells, they would fit across a pencil eraser. Under a microscope, a bacterium can look like a ball, a rod, or a spiral. Bacteria are the dominant living creatures on Earth and they can survive in almost any climate, including in the Yellowstone hot springs, under Antarctic ice, or in the human digestive tract. It has been estimated that there are 5×10^{30} (a nonillion) bacteria on Earth, which accounts for much of the Earth's biomass, more than that of all plants and animals combined.

Sometimes people talk about only bacteria when they talk about the human microbiome, but other life forms are there too, it's just that they are a little easier to overlook. Fungi and viruses don't make up as big a piece of the pie and they aren't as widely studied as bacteria. So are other, even smaller, bugs that we are learning more about all the time.[2] Viruses are ultra-small infectious agents that replicate inside of other cells. You know about cold viruses, and there are others that live in the mouth, such as the herpes virus. Beyond human viruses, there are viruses that attack bacteria. Wherever bacteria are, so go bacteriophages; these bacteria-infecting viruses outnumber bacteria, humans, whales, trees, and everything else put together.[3]

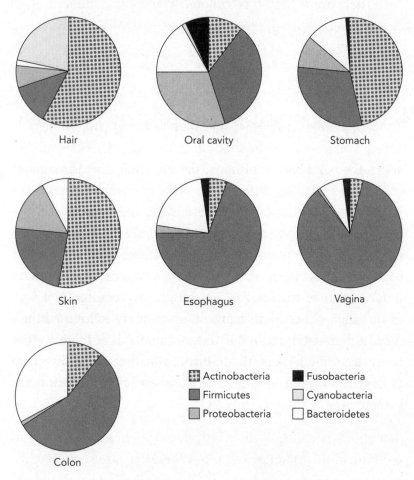

Figure 1.1: Bacterial composition in different microbiomes of the human body.

Fungi, such as mushrooms and yeast, have a different cellular makeup than animals or plants. Certain fungi thrive in the human body, contributing to the microbiome. You have probably heard of fungal infections causing vaginal yeast infections, jock itch, or athlete's foot. Still, bacteria make up the large majority of the microbiome.

There are at least 100 trillion bacteria living in the human intestinal tract, and taken together they have at least 100 times as many genes as our own genome.[4]

There are big microbiomes and then there are small microbiomes. When we talk about the human microbiome, we are talking about the compilation of *all* of the bugs that live throughout the whole body. Each particular place in the body may have its own specific microbiome. There is the oral microbiome, the gut microbiome, the vaginal microbiome, the skin microbiome, the urinary tract microbiome, and the list goes on and on. It's a universe that we are only beginning to explore. Each of these unique areas of the body has a distinctive community of bacteria, fungi, viruses, and more. In ecology, we call it a "niche." A niche is an environment with a certain set of conditions that favors a certain kind of life. In turn, the lifeforms can affect the environment. We will talk more about ecological niches when we tour the mouth in Chapter 3.

YOUR GOOD BUGS

One reason I call it the "magnificent" microbiome is because it does so many good things for us. Let's start with the bacteria in the gut, which we know so much about. Bacteria in your gut make vitamins that you need for blood clotting and metabolism, vitamin K and biotin.[5] They "talk" to your immune system to tell it how to respond—they can tell it to calm down or ramp up an attack. They can soothe and calm down angry, inflamed tissue. Bacteria help to keep a strong barrier between your gut and bloodstream, which protects you from disease. Your microbiota help you get nutrients and calories from your food, and they fine-tune your metabolism. But perhaps the most important role of your good bacteria is that *they protect you from infection*. They serve as a biological defense against bad bugs that might want to invade and cause disease.

On the flip side, when your gut bacteria are out of balance, it can cause obesity, nutritional deficiencies, inflammatory bowel disease, autoimmune disease, nervous system disease, asthma, eczema, or cancer. We absolutely, 100 percent, need our good bacteria for optimum health. We would be very sick and weak without these microbes living inside and on us.[6, 7, 8, 9]

Bacteria were on Earth at least
3 billion years before humans.

THE ECOSYSTEMS INSIDE US

Another reason our microbiome is so magnificent is because it is unimaginably complex. Let's use a rainforest ecosystem as an example of how microbial ecology in the body works. In a rainforest, all of the components work together to build a healthy forest ecology that nurtures and sustains life. There are tall trees that need access to the sun. There are shrubs under those trees, which grow much better in shade. There are spots where the bright sun beams down all day, and certain plants grow well there. There is dark, rich soil. There are bacteria and fungi that help chew up old, dead trees and plants and turn them to dirt again. The more plants, trees, animals, and insects that live in this environment, the more diverse it is, and the healthier it is. Biological diversity, or a broad spectrum of different organisms, is often considered to be a sign of a healthy ecosystem.

Each of these special environments with particular characteristics (sun, shade, etc.) is considered an ecological niche, because it hosts a certain type of plant and that plant in turn affects its environment. Ecological niches are central to the field of ecology, and we will talk about them more as we take a tour of the mouth in Chapter 3.

Let's continue this comparison of a rainforest ecological system with the gut microbiome. The gut microbiome is also a specific environment housing a sophisticated community of lifeforms. The gut provides an environment that bugs love: It is rich in nutrition and mucus. The gut thrives with lots of different kinds of bacteria, indicating biological diversity. Some bacteria are in high amounts, some are in low amounts. Some survive better if they live close together with their neighbors. Bacteria produce chemicals that are beneficial to the gut and to the immune system. They make chemicals that other bacteria eat or that repel certain bacteria. To keep the gut microbiome healthy, then, you have to think about it more as an ecological system with communities of bacteria and an environment it depends on. It's wild and wondrous.

THE ORAL MICROBIOME

The microorganisms living in the human oral cavity make up the oral microbiome. It also covers microbes in adjacent areas such as the nose, pharynx, and the upper portions of the esophagus and lungs. The oral microbiome has one of the most diverse bacterial populations in the body, second only to the gut microbiome.[10] You will notice that we often talk about the oral microbiome in the context of the gut microbiome (see page 85). Much of what we know about the microbes that live inside our bodies comes from the research on the gastrointestinal tract microbiota. It's a good jumping-off point, and most of it applies to the oral cavity, as well. It's been a major subject of research and everyone, including me, has been interested and excited about the gut microbiome in recent years.

You are swallowing at least 140 billion bacteria each day, seeding your gastrointestinal tract with the microbes from your mouth.

But, what lies at the beginning of the gut? The mouth and nose. This means that the oral microbiome and the gut microbiome are inextricably linked. What happens in the mouth also happens in the gut. With its critical position at the front entrance to the gastrointestinal tract, your mouth supplies millions of bacteria to your gut every time you swallow!

The gut has gotten the lion's share of the headlines. But the oral microbiome is equally impressive. Amazingly, the oral microbiome influences health or disease in many other systems of the body, not just the gut. The well-documented link between the oral microbiome and heart disease, diabetes, joint disease, and gut health proves that the oral microbiome is ready to take its rightful place on center stage.

Until now, the oral microbiome has been largely forgotten. My goal is to dust off the research on the oral microbiome, bring it to light, and make it easier to understand. That will be the topic of Chapter 5.

In 1890, Willoughby Miller wrote the first book implicating oral bacteria as a cause of tooth decay. Called *Micro-Organisms of the Human Mouth*, it sparked a worldwide movement of toothbrushing and flossing.[11]

THE GUT MICROBIOME

The gut microbiome has been wildly popular in the last ten years, and you have probably heard it mentioned in the news, in books, on the internet, or even when talking with friends. There are books about the gut microbiome and even cookbooks that tell you how to "feed" your magnificent microbiome. Or maybe you have just heard people talking about the drawbacks of antibiotics, which can damage the gut microbiome.

The gut microbiome refers to the microbes living in the gastrointestinal tract. While the gastrointestinal tract officially includes the mouth, pharynx, esophagus, stomach, small intestines, large intestines, and rectum, usually people are talking about microbes living in the small and large intestines when they mention the "gut microbiome."

What started all of this? I would venture to say it was the Human Microbiome Project, initiated by the National Institutes of Health in 2008. They started what seemed like an impossible feat: to characterize the entire human microbiome. Perhaps after sequencing the entire human genome (or the human DNA code), it seemed like a natural next step to figure out what the DNA of our microbiome looked like. I'm sure the scientific community took a collective gasp of anticipation at the thought of exploring and identifying all the microbes that colonize the human body! It was no small undertaking.

The gut microbiome and oral microbiome have so many similarities that I refer to them as "kissing cousins," and you will see my reasoning in Chapter 7. Much of what you learn about the oral microbiome in this book can be applied to the gut microbiome, as well.

An Unlikely Pregnancy Test

Gracie visited her dental hygienist, Margaret, for her regular cleaning. Margaret had taken care of Gracie's teeth many times over the years. She noticed that Gracie's gums looked different this time. They were rolled, swollen, and puffy. Margaret asked Gracie if she was on her period, as hormonal shifts could sometimes cause these changes. Gracie said no.

Margaret asked if she was about to start her period. Again, Gracie said that it wasn't the case. Margaret said, "Well, from the standpoint of your gums, it looks like you could be pregnant." They carried on through the dental cleaning without another mention of it. One week later, Margaret got a call from Gracie. She told her, "You were right! I *am* pregnant!" Margaret had predicted Gracie's pregnancy even before the typical pregnancy tests. And Gracie's story of finding out she was pregnant at the dentist's office made it into her newborn's baby book, too.

The Human Microbiome Project studied the microbes in 300 healthy people to figure out what bugs were there, what they were doing, and how they differed from one person to another. After figuring out what a "healthy microbiome" looked like, they could move on to study how the microbiome changes with certain diseases, such as inflammatory bowel disease or diabetes.

One thing that was so special about this project is it used the most cutting-edge technology available, a method called quantitative polymerase chain reaction (qPCR) that identifies microbes based on their DNA code. Just like sequencing the human genome launched us into a whole new realm of exploration and scientific understanding, so did characterizing the DNA of the microbes that live on and in us. With this technique, the number of bacteria that we could identify skyrocketed.

Historically, we have identified bacteria based on *if* and *how* they grow in a petri dish. These bacteria are usually taken from a blood, stool, or urine culture. It worked for many, many years, and clinical laboratories still diagnose infections based on this technique. But it has flaws. The biggest flaw is that it misses bacteria that don't like to grow in artificial conditions. DNA methods like those used in the Human Microbiome Project made it possible to see 50 percent more microbes than had ever been seen before.[12, 13, 14] This was a tremendous success and fundamentally changed our understanding of the human microbiome forever!

WHAT TO EXPECT IN THIS BOOK

In this book, we will explore the magnificent oral microbiome and how keeping it in balance can promote health from head to toe. We will tour the oral cavity, get familiar with the immune system that defends the mouth, and review the most common oral diseases that crop up when the oral microbiome is out of balance. We will review the evidence about oral health and natural, safe things you can do to optimize your oral microbiome. The oral microbiome is the next big thing since the gut microbiome, and you'll find out why keeping your oral microbiome healthy can lower your risk of heart disease, stomach ulcers, rheumatoid arthritis, diabetes, and even lower your blood pressure.

Takeaways

- You are made up of at least as many microbial cells as human cells, and probably more.

- Your "good bugs" promote health and ward off disease.

- The bacteria, viruses, fungi, and other microscopic organisms that live inside and on your body make up your microbiome.

- The gut microbiome is diverse and complex, like a tropical rainforest.

- The Human Microbiome Project led the way in microbiome research.

- The oral microbiome and gut microbiome are inextricably linked.

CHAPTER 2

DYSBIOSIS, INFECTION, AND PROTECTION

*"I grew up on antibiotics. Every ailment—
sore throats, earaches, flus—warranted
a trip to the doctor and in most cases
some kind of prescription."*

—Carré Otis, model and actress

Your microbiome contains bugs that protect and benefit you, and it contains bugs that can harm you. Remember that by "bugs," I mean the bacteria, fungi, and viruses that make up your microbiota. Less than 1 percent of microorganisms can harm you. The other 99 percent do no harm and may even improve your health.[15]

Microbiology and medicine have historically concentrated on the bugs that harm us, also called pathogens. These are the big, bad bugs that can create disease and make us miserable. However, amidst all of the fanfare about the bad bugs, everyone overlooked the good bugs. You've heard the saying "One bad apple spoils the bunch"? Well, the bad bugs have given *all* of the bugs in our microbiome a bad rap. Even the bugs that are beneficial or harmless to us have been swept up with the bad opinion we have of bacteria.

I want you to learn in this book that bad bugs are the minority. They can't do any damage if you have strong, healthy levels of good bugs. And the strategy for the future, in this great age of understanding the microbiome, is to promote and nourish your good bugs instead of trying to kill the bad ones.

Your beneficial microbiota protect you from pathogens, make vitamins, regulate your immune response, and can even help you lose weight. But most importantly, they form a living resistance against infection by bad bugs. I like to imagine an endless line of little bacterial soldiers, standing shoulder to shoulder, physically preventing enemy bacteria from penetrating their lines. In Chapter 5, we will dive into more detail about the microbes that call our mouths home. But first, let's talk about the relationship between good bugs and bad ones.

INFECTION OR PROTECTION?

We are exposed to many bad bugs all day, every day. But when our good bugs are healthy and forming a strong defensive line, the bad bugs cannot wiggle their way through our defenses and create infection. When a pathogen is in high numbers, or if good bugs are weak and provide an opportunity, it can cause an infection.[16] In an infection, a microorganism invades the body's tissues and multiplies, and the body reacts to the infection or to the toxins it makes. Many pathogens make toxins that are harmful to us. Certain disease-causing bacteria, fungi, and parasites can lead to infections. In a healthy person, these infections are short-lived but in a weak or sick person, they can be deadly. However, the other 99 percent of normal bacteria that live in your mouth and your gut do not count as infections, since they are your commensal, or normal, microbiota. Let's look at some of the bad bugs that you probably get exposed to every day, without realizing it.

Salmonella is a pathogenic bacterium that has a bad reputation because even a few cells of it can cause food poisoning and symptoms of diarrhea, vomiting, and fever. It is common in raw meat, poultry, eggs, and washed, ready-to-eat foods like berries, tomatoes, and leafy greens.

Escherichia coli O157 is another common cause of infection or food poisoning we hear about in the news. It's brought on by eating contaminated, undercooked foods such as hamburger meat, lettuce, or spinach. Many, many kinds of *E. coli* are harmless and they naturally live in our bodies as well as those of livestock. However, *E. coli* O157 can cause bloody diarrhea.

Here's the amazing thing: You get exposed to Salmonella and *E. coli* O157 in your daily life via contaminated food, undercooked food, restaurants, contaminated water, sick people handling your food, door handles, bathrooms, etc. These are all sources. Even though you don't have bloody diarrhea or vomiting, you *do* get exposed to these bacteria on a regular basis.

But, your good bugs are doing their jobs. They are preventing *E. coli* O157 and Salmonella and the other bacteria, fungi, and parasites like them from setting up shop and creating infection in your body. Thank you, good bugs!

Of course, on the off chance that you do get food poisoning, it likely means that your defenses are compromised. Either your immune system is down or your microbiome is weakened. In these instances, the bug could easily invade, replicate, and harm you. It can also just be bad luck—a particularly toxic form of a bacteria in high amounts.

DYSBIOSIS

Now that we understand what an infection is, let's talk about dysbiosis. Dysbiosis is a major concept in gut health, oral health, and the human microbiome. Our good bugs are stable and live in harmony with us unless they are disturbed by medicine, disease, low pH (acidity), or major dietary changes.[17] When these bugs are thrown out of balance, it causes dysbiosis.

Just like a tropical rainforest, the microbial community in the mouth (and in the gut) is rich and complex. Millions and billions of bacteria live together in harmony with some competition for resources. Some are growing, some are dying, and most are eating, making waste, and making energy and other by-products. When all your bacteria, fungi, and viruses are living together in balance, without making you sick, but protecting you from outside invaders, your microbiome is in good health.

Dysbiosis is when microbes don't grow enough or when they overgrow from their normal balance, causing you symptoms.

Simply, dysbiosis is imbalance in your microbiome. It's not an infection per se, because it is an unhealthy shift in your microbial communities that can give you symptoms, rather than a single, well-known pathogenic microbe causing infection, like Salmonella or *E. coli* O157.

In dysbiosis, certain bacteria in the community can grow and take over, causing imbalance in the system. When growing out of control, these bugs can produce toxins that harm us, they can irritate the adjacent tissues, and they can activate the immune system. When the wrong bugs start to take over, they can crowd out beneficial bacteria, which opens you up to infections by pathogens. For example, gut dysbiosis can cause gas, bloating, loose stools, or maldigestion, and it can make a person more likely to pick up *Clostridium difficile*, a pathogenic bacterium that causes diarrhea. Oral dysbiosis can cause cavities, gingivitis, root canal infections, or bad breath (Chapter 6). Just like we now understand the power and magnificence of our healthy microbiome, we also need to understand that dysbiosis weakens it and leaves us wide open to disease and infection.

There are a few different types of dysbiosis:[18]

- Insufficient growth of normal microbiota is a type of microbial imbalance that results from *not having enough* good bacteria. This leaves the host open to infection and bacterial overgrowth.

- Loss of microbial diversity is a type of dysbiosis that occurs when you don't have a rich, healthy variety of microorganisms.

- Overgrowth of normal microbiota occurs when normal microbes grow excessively. This can cause mild symptoms or no symptoms at all.

- Overgrowth of potentially harmful organisms does not usually cause a problem, but if given the opportunity, they will rise to power and take over. These microbes can cause symptoms and they can crowd out good bugs. They also may cause no symptoms.

Once you have dysbiosis, it may or may not be easy to fix. In a healthy person who is eating a healthy diet, taking probiotics alone might be enough to tip the scales back to a healthy microbiome. Someone with chronic symptoms may need to consult with a healthcare practitioner to treat their microbial dysbiosis. Even in a healthy person, a single infection could cause dysbiosis and their microbiome may never fully get back to normal. In this situation, a health professional can really help. Clinicians often try to boost beneficial bacteria, wipe out the problem-causing microbes, and then continue rebuilding the good bacteria and strengthening the immune system. We discuss these treatments and how to find a provider in Chapter 9.

WHAT IS "NORMAL"

If your microbiome is made up of all of the normal bugs that inhabit your body, then the make-up of those bugs is your microbial balance. Interestingly, each person's microbiome has its own "setpoint," or homeostasis, and it doesn't match to anyone else's (except maybe to family members living in the same house). So, the composition of your microbiome is unique to *you*. While you and I may carry many of the same kinds of microbes, it's pretty much certain that there will be a lot of differences and we will carry our bugs in different proportions from each other. This has led some researchers to identify groups of bacteria that are common to most of us (called "enterotypes" or a "core microbiome"), which we will discuss more in Chapter 5.

If there is no "optimum" bacterial balance for all of us, it makes it pretty hard to tell someone that their microbiome is healthy or that it's not healthy enough. It also makes it impossible to know what bacterial imbalance, or dysbiosis, looks like for a given individual. But the answer to this riddle is to test your microbiome over time so that you can learn what is normal, or not normal, for you. Testing the microbiome helps us figure out normal bacterial balance, dysbiosis, and infection, although it is still an imperfect science. I will tell you more about how to test your microbial compadres in Chapter 9.

ANTIBIOTICS

Antibiotics are one of the biggest dangers to our microbiomes. These medications transformed medicine 100 years ago, allowing us to live longer lives and to defeat deadly infections.[19] Yay! However, antibiotics have a serious side effect. They wipe out *all* of our bacteria, not just infection-causing bacteria. And while our microbiomes grow back rapidly after we finish antibiotics, they never return to their original stable state.[20] Antibiotics shift bacterial communities and deplete diversity within three or four days of beginning treatment.[21] As you might imagine, cutting down your microbes is a serious crime. These bugs help you make nutrients, prime your immune system, fight and defend against foreign invaders, and tune your metabolism.

Antibiotics should be used with caution, but unfortunately, doctors haven't always been so wise. I grew up in the '80s and '90s. My sister, brother, and I had regular ear infections growing up, so there was usually a bottle of bubble gum–flavored antibiotics—amoxicillin—in the refrigerator (Yummy! Not.) Antibiotics were prescribed when there were ear infections, colds, and sore throats. We now know that these were not good reasons to take antibiotics, because these ailments are not always caused by a bacterial infection. Research shows that 50 percent of antibiotics prescribed at doctors' offices are unnecessary.[22] And 30 to 60 percent of antibiotics prescribed in the intensive care unit of the hospital are unnecessary or inappropriate.

In 2010, there were enough antibiotic prescriptions written in the United States to give every single American one dose.

On a bigger scale, something much graver and more dangerous than pathogenic bacteria has emerged from overuse of antibiotics: antibiotic-resistant bacteria. These are superbugs that cannot be destroyed with antibiotics. Take the pathogens we talked about earlier as an example: These are bugs that can cause infections in people and have unwanted effects like diarrhea, vomiting, and fever. Now, give those bugs antibiotics for a short time. The medication will kill most of the pathogenic bacteria, but not all. Any bacterial survivors are likely resistant to the antibiotic. It's Darwinian natural selection.

Bacteria are very adaptable. They grow and multiply lightning-fast. They also can easily share their DNA with each other to help their survival. If you try to kill a bacterial infection a few times unsuccessfully, you are slowly cultivating a pathogen that can resist the antibiotic. This is why the doctor will now tell you to take *all* of your antibiotics for the full duration of the prescription, even after your symptoms have gone away. If you stop early, then you are just training certain bacteria how to withstand antibiotics. If you apply this strategy of prescribing lots of unnecessary antibiotics to large human populations (like in hospital settings) over decades, you have essentially bred a highly dangerous superbug that can't be destroyed with antibiotics.

> *"When antibiotics first came out, nobody could have imagined we'd have the resistance problem we face today. We didn't give bacteria credit for being able to change and adapt so fast."*
> —Bonnie Bassler, molecular biology professor and chair, Princeton University

See Chapter 9 for treatments to help your microbiome bounce back when you have no other choice but to take antibiotics. "Herbal antibiotics" can help remove infections and don't have the same tendency of creating antibiotic-resistant superbugs.

Takeaways

- Infections are caused by microbes that invade the body, multiply, and cause a reaction, including illness.

- Dysbiosis is a state of microbial imbalance: either too few or too many bugs. It can also cause illness.

- Good bugs are your number one defense against infection and dysbiosis.

- Antibiotics kill infections but also kill good bugs.

- Antibiotic overuse has created drug-resistant superbugs.

CHAPTER 3

A TOUR OF
THE MOUTH

*"The first thing I do in the morning is brush
my teeth and sharpen my tongue."*
—Dorothy Parker, American writer

In this chapter, we will learn why the mouth is ideally suited for its microbial residents and how it influences the rest of the body. The mouth's strategic location has immediate impacts on the immune system and on the gut microbiome. But aside from its prime location, the mouth has special qualities that appeal to the oral microbiome. One of those qualities is a constant flow of saliva, which washes away bacteria, carries food, and helps good bugs latch on to teeth. And you might think your gums, cheeks, tongue, and teeth have a lot in common, but your bacteria would beg to differ. In fact, each of these areas in the mouth caters to a different group of bacteria. Overall, the mouth is uniquely located at the headwaters of the GI tract, has a number of specialized habitats for bacteria, and is dependent on saliva. These are only some of the reasons that 20 billion bugs have taken up residence in our mouths!

LOCATION, LOCATION, LOCATION

One of the most important things about the mouth is its location. The mouth is uniquely situated at the front entrance of the body and the beginning of the gastrointestinal tract and lungs. That makes it the first point of entry for anything from the outside world. Indeed, there is a constant stream of foreign organisms into the mouth. Therefore, the immune system in the mouth has to be fierce and vigilant. It has to carefully and effectively differentiate good guys from bad. It has to attack and destroy harmful outsiders but welcome friendly outsiders. We are talking about identifying foods, water, minerals, vitamins, bacteria, fungi, parasites, toxins, and more. This is not a job for the faint of heart. It's tough work. In Chapter 4, we will explore the incredible immune system that keeps us safe and in a state of harmony.

The mouth shares its immune system and its general architecture with the whole digestive tract. The digestive tract includes the mouth, esophagus, stomach, small intestine, large intestines, and rectum. The mouth and the gut are essentially just two different stops on the same bus line, so they have *a lot* in common. Seventy percent of your immune system lives in your gut, specifically in the gut mucosa.[23] Both the mouth and the gut are lined with a mucous membrane. This membrane acts as a physical barrier—a wall—to keep bad stuff out of the bloodstream. Later in this chapter, we will find out what the mucous membrane is made of, and in Chapters 7 and 8, we will discuss why it is crucial to a smart immune system, a healthy body, and low levels of inflammation.

WHAT'S IN A MOUTH?

Let's take a quick tour of the mouth since it's the home of the oral microbiome. Trust me, it's pretty cool. There is so much more going on in there than you ever realized!

The mouth has two types of surfaces. You can feel them with your tongue right now. We have the oral mucosa, also known as the epithelial lining of the mouth, which is soft. Feel the inside of your cheek, your gums, the roof of your mouth, and the floor of your mouth. Those are mucous membranes. These cells turn over regularly, meaning old cells die and new ones grow constantly. Then we have the teeth, which are hard surfaces that are durable and unchanging (or so it seems to the naked eye).

The Barrier

The mucosal barrier is our defensive line. It is incredibly critical to our health and defense. This applies to the mucosal barrier not just in the mouth but throughout the gastrointestinal tract and beyond. Imagine if you didn't have your skin as a barrier between your body and the outside world—you would be wide open to attack and infection. In the same way, your mouth lining is the barrier between the bloodstream and the constant stream of bacteria, food, and chemicals that comes into your mouth.

Therefore, a strong and healthy barrier is an excellent way to keep your mouth healthy.

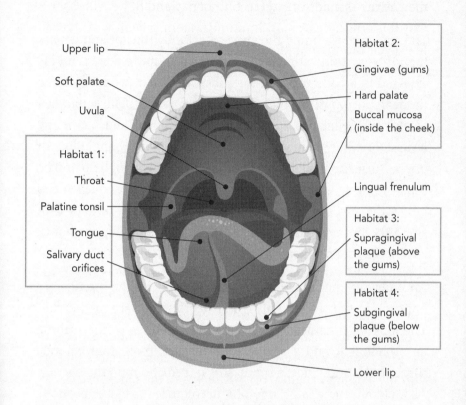

Figure 3.1: Anatomy of the mouth and different habitats for oral microbiota.

Mucous membranes line cavities or cover the surface of organs. They are made of one or more layers of a special type of cells called epithelial cells. Epithelial cells form a flexible, soft, and firm sheet of tissue that wraps around the framework of our organs and cavities. Underneath the sheet of epithelial cells is a type of connective tissue called the lamina propria, which is like cartilage, as well as blood and lymph vessels. Our gums are essentially a layer of cartilage topped by a layer of epithelial tissue, which together cover the jawbone and surround our teeth snugly. This may sound complicated, but it's really just like your skin, only it's on the inside, and it's slimy. Other mucous membranes line the lungs, nose, vagina, esophagus, and of course, the entire gastrointestinal tract. Cool design!

The oral mucosa lining the gums is actually thicker and denser than the gastrointestinal mucosa. It is also more porous and is exposed to a wide range of microbes and their products.[24] The tissue in the mouth is officially described as stratified, squamous (scaly) epithelial tissue because it is flattened and has many layers. Just like your skin, the oral mucosa can handle lots of use because the thick layers of cells on top will slough off and be replaced by new layers that are constantly being produced deep below the surface. Mucin, also known as mucus, or snot (not so pretty, but now you know exactly what we're talking about), covers the oral mucosa.

Another unique thing about the barrier in the mouth, as opposed to that in the gut, is that teeth penetrate the barrier. The mucous membrane on the gums surrounds teeth, forming an attachment and a seal. However, each tooth that extends through the oral mucosa represents *a weak point* in the barrier. As we'll talk about later, microbiota colonize the teeth above the gumline and below the gumline, which mean that bacteria in our mouths are privy to the bloodstream.

That's right. Despite this formidable barrier, bacteria from our mouths regularly get into our bloodstream. The oral mucosa is a "selectively permeable" barrier at best. While it does block many bad things from entry, it also lets a lot of things through, and sometimes it lets in too much. It has been shown that simply brushing your teeth or eating can lead to a surge of bacteria in your bloodstream, called "bacteremia." This process may explain why oral health is intimately tied to the health of the heart, joints, and metabolism. We will discuss this further in Chapter 8.

Your Pearly Whites

Teeth are the hardest tissue in the body and are uniquely able to handle lots of wear, tear, and harsh conditions, such as high acid. There's more than meets the eye when it comes to your sparkling whites. Your teeth are made of enamel, cementum, and pulp-dentine complex. Enamel is that ultra-hard, pretty, white surface on the crowns of your teeth. It is resistant to the acids we eat and the microbiota living in our mouths. Cementum is like enamel because it also coats the tooth, except it coats the *roots* of the tooth.

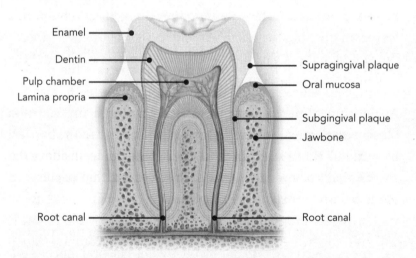

Figure 3.2: The pulp chamber at the center of the tooth contains nerves and a blood supply. Every tooth has a direct line into the bloodstream, which could explain why problems in the mouth can show up in the heart or joints.

As you can see in Figure 3.2, underneath the layer of enamel and cementum is dentin, which makes up most of the tooth. Dentin is composed of 10 percent water, 20 percent type 1 collagen, and 70 percent minerals. Specifically, dentin is mostly a blend of calcium, phosphorus, oxygen, and hydrogen called hydroxy-apatite, which is the fundamental *hard* ingredient in teeth and bones. It's like cement. Additionally, small percentages of magnesium, potassium, and sodium can be found in teeth. Fluorine is also found in teeth, primarily through water fluoridation, fluoride treatments, and toothpaste.[25]

One of the cool things about teeth and bones is that they are always under construction. Inside the dentin, teeth are constantly being broken down and rebuilt by "construction worker" cells, called osteoclasts and osteoblasts. This goes for bone as well. If you needed a super-strong bridge, wouldn't you always have to maintain it? The result is a very strong and resilient hard tissue to chomp your food with. However, when teeth are broken down at a faster rate than they are getting rebuilt, this leaves an opening for microbes to damage the tooth further.[26] We will talk about this more when we discuss cavities and the oral microbiome in Chapter 6.

At the very center of each tooth is pulp, where you can find blood vessels and nerves. Do you remember when you lost a baby tooth? Remember that hole on the underside/inside of the tooth? That's where pulp would normally be. If you've ever had tooth pain or sensitivity, that's because the pulp of the tooth was involved. Pulp acts like an alarm system for the tooth. It will tell you when there is a problem. Pulp contains blood vessels and nerves and osteoblasts, which make dentin. Each tooth has a line into the bloodstream via the pulp, meaning that the teeth are well connected to the whole body. It's called the pulp-dentine complex because these two neighboring tissues work together closely to create the hard structure of teeth and keep them healthy.

Teeth are the hardest tissues in the body and are uniquely able to handle lots of wear, tear, and harsh conditions such as high acid.

THE ECOSYSTEMS INSIDE US

I wouldn't bore you with all of these details except that each of these areas in the mouth harbors *different* microbiota. Those little buggers are picky. Some live best in and on the throat, tonsils, saliva, and tongue. Other microbes live on the inside of the cheeks, the roof of the mouth (the hard palate), and gums (also known as the gingivae). There are whole communities of bugs that live on the teeth *above* the gumline, which are quite different from the bugs that live on the teeth *below* the gumline. The microbiota living in our mouths colonize all of these areas.

The reason we need to know a little about the anatomy of the mouth is because the bugs in our mouths like each of these areas for specific reasons. For example, the teeth don't shed cells, so they are easier for microbes to hang on to. And the bugs that live under the gumline die if they get too much oxygen; they prefer to be buried, so that air can't reach them.

A study of the oral microbiome showed that each of these areas is a distinct ecological niche. Despite being so close in proximity, very different bacterial communities colonize these sites:

- Throat, tonsils, saliva, and tongue

- Gums, cheeks, and roof of the mouth

- Supragingival plaque on teeth (microbes above the gumline)

- Subgingival plaque on teeth (microbes below the gumline)

Each of these areas in our mouths represents an ecological niche that, because of its unique characteristics, attracts and fosters the growth of particular communities of bacteria. An ecological niche is a fundamental concept in ecology and describes a relationship between a species and its environment. In an ecological niche, a species both shapes and is shaped by its environment. This hearkens back to Chapter 1, where we compared the microbiome to a biodiverse rainforest. Some plants like the sun, some like the shade, and some are in between. A rainforest has ecological niches that can support all of them. So does the mouth provide ecological niches to different types of bacteria that can then set up shop and call them home.

A SEA OF SALIVA

Amidst all of these different "ecological niches," which I'm sure you never knew were in your mouth, is a sea of saliva. That, I'm sure, you *did* know about! Saliva is your best friend, believe it or not. It is absolutely vital for your mouth to stay healthy. Saliva controls the pH, or the acid-base balance, in your mouth by constantly keeping the calcium and phosphate levels high. Too much acid can damage teeth. Calcium and phosphate make the pH more basic, which helps build and repair healthy teeth (a process called mineralization) and wards off tooth damage and break-down.[27] When the pH is just right, nutrient minerals like calcium and phosphorus can be formed into bones and teeth.

Saliva is packed with substances that protect you from unfriendly microbes and help to balance your microbiome. Saliva contains an enzyme called lysozyme, which defends you from bacteria by breaking down their cell walls. Enzymes are worker proteins that catalyze reactions, or change molecules in the body by acting on them. Saliva contains another enzyme called lactoperoxidase, which is antibacterial, antiviral, antifungal, and antiparasitic. It just so happens to help prevent cavities, gingivitis, and periodontal disease. Lactoferrin is a protein found in saliva, as well as breastmilk, that steals nutrients from bacteria as a way of starving them out. And saliva contains immune system proteins called immunoglobulins that bind up and eliminate bad stuff like pathogens or foreign food molecules that might be harmful. The immune defenses in the saliva are immunoglobulins A, G and M (IgA, IgG, and IgM for short).

Saliva supplies nutrition to the microbes in your mouth. It contains proline-rich glycoproteins (sugar-protein molecules) that help bacteria anchor to teeth. On the other hand, saliva cleans your mouth and washes bacteria off of your teeth. You might think of this as a continuous "trimming of the hedges." While saliva makes it possible for bacteria to attach and live on teeth, it also continually washes over bacteria, freeing up some to be swallowed. Because bacteria are constantly shed from surfaces in the mouth, the saliva carries a lot of bacteria and is even a good specimen for measuring a person's oral microbiome.[28, 29]

Each milliliter of saliva (roughly ¼ teaspoon)
contains 140 million bacterial cells!
The average person makes around a liter
of saliva each day, which would come to
140 billion bacterial cells in saliva each day.

THERE'S NO PLACE LIKE HOME

The mouth is a unique place and that's why microbes love it. There's plenty of food, a steady flow of saliva, and specialized habitats that appeal to their needs. There is a soft, flexible sheet of tissue called the epithelium that forms the mucous membranes in the mouth, which also serves as a physical barrier and immune system launching pad, making it critically important to our health. So, given what we learned about the layout and topography of the oral cavity in this chapter, we can move on to talk about the audacious immune system that walks a tightrope between attack and tolerance and how our good bugs help it do just that.

Takeaways

- The mouth is positioned at the entrance to the GI tract and is the first meeting place between your immune system and the outside world.

- The oral cavity has at least four different ecological niches that host different microbiota.

- A soft, flexible membrane of epithelial cells, called the oral mucosa, lines the oral cavity.

- The oral mucosa creates a physical barrier between the bloodstream and a constant stream of microorganisms in the mouth.

- Saliva fosters your oral microbiome by supplying nutrients, helping microbes attach to surfaces, and destroying enemy microbes.

CHAPTER 4

HAIL TO THE IMMUNE SYSTEM

"The most powerful therapeutic in the world is our own immune system."

—Francis deSouza, American entrepreneur

Remember, the mouth is the gateway to the entire gastrointestinal tract. It's the front entrance. You don't leave your front door unlocked, do you? You need protection at the front of your home so that only people you choose can enter. Likewise, the mouth is equipped with defenses to protect the body from potentially harmful outside invaders. However, most of what comes into the mouth is not dangerous: It's mainly food, water, pollen, friendly bacteria, friendly fungi, etc. So, the immune system has to figure out who is a bad guy and who is a good guy.

AN EPIC GAME OF "WHERE'S WALDO?"

The immune system is incredible. I liken its job to the Where's Waldo? book series. The exercise in these books was to comb through huge crowds of people to find Waldo, a single quirky guy wearing red-and-white stripes and a hat. Likewise, the immune system has to find Waldo, in this case a pathogenic "bad guy," and make sure all of the defenses are up wherever Waldo may try to gain entry. On the other hand, the immune system has to ignore *everyone else* who is totally harmless—the good and neutral microbes. And the immune system has to remember who is who, over time, without making mistakes. This is no easy job.

There are two major branches of immune function at the mucous membrane, and they have to work together. The first line of defense is called the innate immune system because humans have evolved it over millennia. The second branch is the adaptive immune system (also called the acquired immune system). As the name implies, this is the part of the immune system that can learn as it goes. It has a memory. When you get exposed to a new thing, your adaptive immune system can remember whether it is a good guy or a bad guy.

Your immune system operates within an infrastructure of base camps and superhighways that make up the lymphatic system. Lymph tissues include lymph nodes, tonsils, and other tissues and organs that fight infections in the body. This is how the body delivers immune-fighting cells from the tops of our heads to the tips of our toes. Mucosa-associated lymphoid tissue (MALT) is the immune system network that monitors and protects the mucosal surfaces of the body. If the mouth lining, or epithelium, is the frontline of the battle, the MALT act as the headquarters where immune "soldiers" congregate, get their orders, and head back out to battle. The tonsils, salivary glands, and adenoids are the principal MALTs in the oral cavity.[30] In the gut, these headquarters are called gut-associated lymphoid tissue (GALT), and in the nose it is called naso-pharynx associated lymphoid tissue (NALT).[31] Lymph nodes are other major basecamps in the infection-fighting network. They are knots in the net of lymphatic vessels. Each lymph node is filled with immune cells called lymphocytes. They act like filtering stations to purify the lymph before it enters the bloodstream. Lymph nodes are the prime sites where immune cells congregate, get orders, grow their armies, and head back out to the tissues to continue protecting and defending. Lymph is a clear fluid that irrigates our bodies, supplying us with immune fighter cells and keeping our body fluids in balance.

THE INNATE IMMUNE SYSTEM AND THE BARRIER

The innate immune system is somewhat straightforward, perhaps because it is so ancient. It has evolved over millennia. It acts as the first line of defense against threats and recognizes foreign invading microbes and destroys them. But before we get into how the innate immune system eliminates the enemy, let's take a minute to recognize the physical barrier itself.

The first part of our innate immune defenses in the mouth is the physical barrier itself, the oral mucosa. The mucosal barrier has to keep bad stuff out but let the good stuff in. For instance, it is responsible for keeping disease-causing microorganisms out but letting food and nutrients in. It also has to let beneficial microbiota hang around. This is a delicate balance to uphold. As we discussed in Chapter 3, the cells in the oral mucosa are flattened and lined up, one over another, to form a continuous sheet of tissue that is hard to penetrate, yet porous. It is thicker and denser that the gastrointestinal mucosa but nevertheless still permeable and fragile. The mucous membrane is also coated in a dense layer of mucin, or snot. The barrier is also covered with saliva, which contains immunoglobulins, antimicrobial proteins, and enzymes that can ward off bad guys.[32]

Meanwhile, the innate immune system is ready to pounce. It uses proteins called Toll-like receptors to look for unwelcome microorganisms. Toll-like receptors stick out of the epithelial lining into the mouth and fish for suspicious foreign invaders. Dendritic cells, a type of immune cell, sit on the oral mucosa and project their little fingers, called dendrites, into the oral cavity. Dendritic cells take samples, recognize microbes, and report them back to headquarters (launching an immune response through the adaptive immune system's T cells, which we will discuss next).[33] Other innate immune cells include natural killer cells, macrophages, neutrophils, eosinophils, and basophils. These cells basically eat the bad guys or release toxic bombs to destroy them.

THE ADAPTIVE IMMUNE SYSTEM

The adaptive immune system is responsible for eliminating bad bacteria, viruses, tumors, and parasites. It also tells the body to tolerate harmless foods and microbes, or see certain foods as dangerous (for example, food allergies). Adaptive immunity is a slower response than innate immunity but has the benefit of being able to adapt to whatever new and unusual threats come our way. Even better: It remembers its enemies, so if they try to come around again, they are easily eliminated.

The Immune System in the Mouth and in the Gut

So many things about the mouth and the gut are similar, including the architecture and the immune defenses. The epithelial lining of the intestines is nearly identical to that in the oral cavity, and since so much more is known about the gastrointestinal mucosa, it serves as a model to understand the mucosal lining elsewhere in the body, including the mouth.[34] One slight difference is that the epithelial lining in the gut has only one layer of cells, whereas the oral mucosa has multiple layers. The MALT in the mouth is very similar to its corollary in the gut, the GALT. Have you heard that 70 percent of your immune system lives in your gut? They are talking about the GALT, or the immune system tissue found at the gut lining. So, everything that we discussed earlier regarding the innate immune system and the adaptive immune system in the mouth applies to the gut as well. The entire mucosal surface of the gastrointestinal tract, starting with the *mouth*, is heavily armed with infection-fighting superhighways and headquarters.

In the mouth, when foreign molecules (antigens) bind to the mucosa, they go through an assembly line–like process during which the adaptive immune system decides on a response. The immune system has three levels of staff: guards, headquarters, and combat soldiers. First, guards in the MALT such as dendritic cells or M cells sample all of the stuff coming into the mouth. Dendritic cells can either recognize a harmless outsider and tolerate it or they can recognize a harmful invader and launch an attack. If they detect a bad guy, dendritic cells at the headquarters of the MALT then tell the combat cells, T and B lymphocytes (T and B cells, for short), to replicate themselves, then stalk and destroy the antigens. T cells attack dangerous cells while B cells clean up the hallways and alleyways between cells. In other words, B cells help keep the space between cells clear of bad guys. B cells produce antibodies specific to each foreign invader. Antibodies are proteins that tag a harmful invader by perfectly binding to it like a lock and key. Once an invader is tagged, the immune system can neutralize or dispose of it. Antibodies help spread the word about bad guys far and wide. Immune cells can communicate all of this information with the help of proteins called cytokines, which can either encourage or discourage attack and inflammation.

In this way, the immune system records a biochemical memory, or imprint, that perfectly identifies the antigen and can be communicated throughout the body so that the antigen is destroyed and never allowed to enter the body—and if it does, it can't get very far. This is a huge over-simplification of the immune system, so please do further reading on this fascinating topic if your interest is piqued.

As you can see, the immune system is armed and dangerous. And if the immune system unleashed its fury on the human body, it would be brutal. So, there are checks and balances in place to control the immune system. Regulatory T cells, sometimes called Treg cells, dampen the aggressive actions of the other T cells. They can even kill aggressive T cells. Treg cells actually calm down the immune system and teach it tolerance. This helps pull the reins on the innate and adaptive immune responses so they don't overreact and harm the host.[35] If Treg cells are defective, autoimmune diseases, allergic diseases, and inflammation can spiral out of control.[36]

Another important immune tool is found in your mouth. Your saliva is loaded with secretory IgA (sIgA), an immunoglobulin produced by B cells in the oral mucosa. It helps trap and eliminate foreign invaders by binding to them, and keeps them from penetrating the oral mucosa or getting into the bloodstream. When something new arrives in the mouth, this component of your adaptive immune system tells everyone else in the neighborhood. It even makes sure that signals are sent downstream so that the gut mucosa can make sIgA antibodies against the new foreigner, too—the oral mucosa helps inform the gut mucosa what is to come.[37] This illustrates that the oral immune system is closely connected with the gut immune system. They are two stops on the same bus line, after all!

The Microbes and the Immune System Do a Dance

Remember the game of "Where's Waldo?" that the immune system is so good at? Here is the other side of the coin. Aside from pinpointing, attacking, and eradicating the bad guys forever, the immune system has to identify and tolerate (or ignore) the good guys. Enter your normal, healthy oral microbiota.

These are microbes that the immune system has worked out an agreement with. They are allowed to hang around. Some of the microbiota actually send signals that tell the immune system to calm down and look the other way. Others stimulate the immune system and help it improve its surveillance. Regulatory T cells are part of the adaptive immune system and promote tolerance, as mentioned earlier.

The oral microbiome can suppress the body's immune reaction or stimulate and "prime" it. Microbial populations have also worked out ways to evade the immune system so that they can hang around without being bothered. It is generally believed that commensal bacteria keep inflammation in the gut and mouth to a minimum. In a healthy mouth, pro-inflammatory and anti-inflammatory mechanisms are kept in check. Certain oral commensal microbiota may affect this balance by decreasing inflammatory cell messages, promoting anti-inflammatory regulatory T cells, or activating immune cells.

Good bacteria can act like anti-inflammatory agents and can promote tolerance. We don't fully understand all of the ways that they do this. However, one of the strongest lines of evidence is that when mice don't have any good bacteria, they develop food allergies. Good bacteria, therefore, educate the immune system so that it doesn't mistakenly attack harmless foods.[38]

Lactobacillus species, a friendly bacteria found in probiotic supplements, can calm down immune messages and ramp up anti-inflammatory chemical messages. Up to 30 to 40 percent of Streptococcus species from the tongue and dental plaque can "scare off" immune cells that are attracted to the gums, thereby protecting their communities from attack.[39]

All of this, and nothing to mention of their role in preventing invasion and infection! I think it's fair to say that good bacteria are partners with the "superorganism" immune system, if not officially part of it. As mentioned in Chapter 1, humans together with our microbial inhabitants are considered "superorganisms." Good bacteria block out or prevent colonization by bad bugs for us each and every day. Remember, this is one of the most important services our little critters do for us.

INFLAMMATION

All of these incredible mechanisms that defend and protect us contribute to our overall levels of inflammation. I think of it as chemical and biological warfare. Inflammation in small doses is very healthy and keeps us in tip-top shape. The immune response needed to kill a pathogen is vital to our survival. Yes, you feel bad when you get sick, but your immune system is going hog-wild eliminating the culprit. In the process, the immune system fires off ammunition to kill the enemy, which causes inflammation, pain, and fever, among other symptoms. But the result is to successfully get rid of the bad guy and never have trouble with him ever again (the immune system has a memory, as we discussed in The Adaptive Immune System starting on page 40).

When inflammation is excessive, however, we have a whole other type of problem. Chronic inflammation suggests that the immune system is overreacting. The innate and adaptive immune systems are super powerful and potent. They don't mess around. So if they unleash their fury for the wrong reason or for an extended period of time, they are very harmful.

Inflammation is a major feature of periodontal disease, heart disease, Crohn's disease, ulcerative colitis, and more. We are going to talk more about inflammatory diseases in Chapters 6, 7, and 8. Just remember that chronic inflammation speaks to a problem with the immune system and the natural processes that are intended to defend and protect us from invasion.

Periodontal disease is an example of the immune system trying to aggressively eradicate certain oral microbiota, but in the process, it seriously damages the host. It unleashes all of its power in the form of tons of immune cells to the gums. Some of the microbes in periodontal disease have learned how to evade the immune system—it essentially stands around, huffing and puffing, trying to find the little buggers. But it never gives up, and eventually, all of the inflammation it has created trying to kill the dental plaque instead destroys the gums and bones surrounding the tooth. We will talk about periodontal disease and dysbiosis in Chapter 6.

LEAKY MOUTH

The importance of the epithelium as a mechanical barrier between the outside and inside world cannot be overstated. A healthy mucosal barrier is absolutely vital for a healthy immune system. If you are interested in gut health, immune health, or the gut microbiome, then you have probably heard of the concept of leaky gut, or intestinal barrier permeability. This is a hypothesis that has come from medical research on the gastrointestinal mucosa.

Leaky gut is a central theory in certain medical and research fields that greatly contributes to our understanding of autoimmune and chronic inflammatory diseases. The gastrointestinal tract has a mucous membrane just like the one in the mouth. The gut mucosa serves as a barrier between the outside world and the bloodstream. Just like the mouth, it is populated with immune cells, immune tissue, and billions of microbes. When the barrier is broken down or damaged, it becomes permeable. Little nicks and holes form in that barrier and then foreign molecules can reach the bloodstream, where they don't belong. This is called intestinal permeability. The reason leaky gut is such an important idea is because it represents a total breakdown of the barrier that protects a person from the outside world. The result is that food, bacteria, fungi, parasites, chemicals, and toxins can get into the bloodstream and set off an even worse kind of immune reaction. The immune system goes on hyperactive red alert and sometimes cannot calm down. Intestinal permeability can increase the risk of chronic inflammatory diseases or autoimmune diseases.[40, 41, 42] Autoimmune diseases are often a case of the immune system getting confused and attacking the tissues of the body instead of the bad guys.

This concept applies to the mouth as well. Remember that the oral mucosa is not an iron-clad barrier. It is porous and selectively permeable. Even in healthy people, the oral mucosa is leaky enough to let bacteria enter the bloodstream, called bacteremia. As we will discuss more in Chapter 8, it means that high levels of bacteria flood into the blood even when we do simple activities like brush our teeth, eat, or get a dental cleaning.

If the barrier in the mouth gets worn down and damaged, then foreign invaders from the outside world would have even easier access to the bloodstream. Bleeding, sore gums, or loose connections between the gums and teeth are a sign of a weak barrier and a "leaky mouth." Remember from Chapter 3 that the oral mucosa has another unique chink in its armor: Every tooth that penetrates the barrier leaves an opening for microbes to enter.

When I was interviewed by Dr. Kara Fitzgerald, a functional medicine practitioner, in 2015, I suggested the idea of leaky mouth. It seemed like a natural next step from leaky gut, which is widely taught in the field of integrative and functional medicine. (Functional medicine is a model of medical treatment that addresses underlying causes of disease to restore each individual to optimum wellness.) Later, I interviewed a functional dentist, Dr. Mary Ellen Chalmers, and learned that she had suggested the same phenomena years earlier. Though leaky mouth is not a recognized condition, it deserves consideration. Leaky mouth could significantly worsen bacteremia. This might explain why and how the health of the oral cavity is so intimately intertwined with the health of the whole body. Stay tuned for more on this in Chapter 8.

IMMUNITY AND THE MOUTH

A constant stream of bacteria and their products makes the mouth vulnerable to invasion from pathogens. The immune system is an incredibly complex network of cells, transport systems, chemical messages, and biological weapons. It operates 24/7 in the background at each mucosal surface of the body. It is intelligent and has a memory. The microbes in the mouth can both stimulate the immune system and suppress it, meaning that the oral microbiome is critical for the development and fine-tuning of the immune system. One of the most important defenses in the mouth is the mucosal barrier itself, which prevents outside invaders from reaching the bloodstream—to a point. The oral mucosa is naturally porous. If this barrier is breached, such as in the form of bleeding gums, leaky mouth could spell trouble for the rest of the body. Lessons from the gut mucosa tell us that this could be the case.

Takeaways

- A constant stream of microbes, chemicals, and toxins make the mouth vulnerable to invasion.

- The oral mucosa is a protective barrier between your body and the outside world.

- The immune system is a complex network of cells, transport systems, chemical messages, and biological weapons that can sort out friend or foe and destroy enemies.

- The oral microbiome can ramp up or calm down the immune response, and is important for fine-tuning the immune system in the mouth.

- Uncontrolled immune reactions and barrier permeability can increase the risk of autoimmune and inflammatory diseases.

- Damage to the oral mucosal barrier, or a leaky mouth, could open up the body to harmful microbes and inflammation.

CHAPTER 5

THE ORAL MICROBIOME

"The mouth houses the second most diverse microbial community in the body."

—Mogens Kilian and colleagues; professor, Department of Biomedicine, Aarhus University, Denmark[43]

In this chapter we will find out where we get our oral microbiome from and who might have a similar one. We will review the benefits of our commensal microbes and why they are so vital to our health. We will talk about Streptococcus, the big bacterial player in the mouth, as well as the Firmicutes and Bacteroidetes phyla, which dominate the gut and the oral microbiomes.

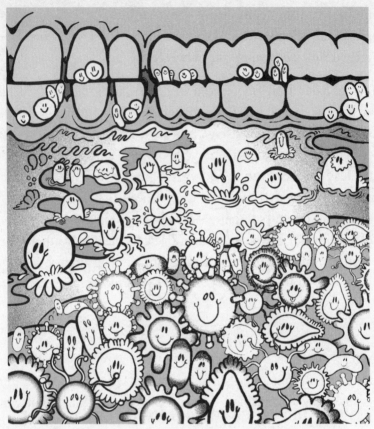

Figure 5.1: Bacteria in the mouth. Both good and bad bacteria live in the mouth, but mostly good.

ORAL MICROBIOTA

Twenty billion bacteria live in your mouth, representing a whopping 770 species. That's nearly three times the Earth's human population. These bacteria thrive in a sea of saliva. There are a number of different microenvironments in the oral cavity where bacteria can grow and make a home. As we discussed earlier, they may live in and on the tongue, throat, tonsils, and saliva; the gums, cheeks, and roof of the mouth; the teeth, above the gumline; and the teeth, below the gumline. Each of these eco-logical niches supports and sustains not just a few bacteria, but huge, complex *communities* of bacteria.

Most of your oral microbiota are normal and healthy. They can improve your health by balancing your immune system, keeping the bad bugs at bay, and helping keep a healthy bar-rier between your mouth and your bloodstream. There are also harmless bacteria, fungi, and viruses in the mouth. They don't necessarily do anything good for you, but they cause no harm either. And of course, there are a few bad bugs lurking around and waiting for a chance to take over and cause trouble. They are often waiting for dysbiosis, or imbalanced microbial com-munities, which gives them a window of opportunity to move in and rise to power. We will learn more about dysbiosis of the oral microbiota and oral pathogens in Chapter 6.

Breakthroughs in DNA analysis led to an explosion of research on the microbiome, and since then, we have discovered count-less new species that had been invisible up to that point. Our older methods of culturing bacteria in a petri dish missed approximately 50 percent of the bugs living in our mouths.[44] We now use molecular methods that identify bacteria based on their genetic code; these are more precise and they don't require that the bug grow in an artificial environment. Even in 2018, the Human Oral Microbiome Database admits that of 770 oral microbiome species we now know of, only 57 percent have names and have been properly characterized.[45] When it comes to the microbes that live in our mouths and influence our whole-body health, we have only scratched the surface.

As a way to organize and understand the tremendous number of bacteria in the world, they are often categorized as aerobic or anaerobic. Aerobic bacteria can live in oxygen. Anaerobic bacteria don't do well (and can die) in oxygen. Anaerobic bacteria tend to be found in deep, dark crevices where the air cannot reach them, such as the gut or on the teeth below the gumline.

Microbiologists also classify the big world of bacteria as gram-negative and gram-positive; this simply describes the cell walls of bacteria. Gram-positive bacteria have a thick cell wall with peptidoglycan and teichoic acids, which will stain purple. Gram-negative bacteria have a thin peptidoglycan layer and will not stain purple. This characterization is a throwback from the days when we couldn't analyze bacteria based on their DNA, only on how they were tested or how they grew in a petri dish on a laboratory bench.

Benefits of the Microbiome

Commensal organisms, or indigenous organisms, are the microbes that naturally colonize our bodies and either benefit us or do no harm. These are the "good guys." You don't want to leave home without them. While we are still in the beginning stages of understanding how commensal microbes benefit our health, it seems that they may help to prevent allergies, eczema, asthma, reflux esophagitis, inflammatory bowel disease, irritable bowel syndrome, psoriasis, obesity, cancer, and cardiovascular disease.[46, 47]

Your commensal microbes protect you from invasion by foreign outsiders that mean to cause you harm. Bad bugs are always around, but with enough good bugs, you are protected. Good bugs work together to promote stability and resilience of the microbiome so that big changes, like those that occur after taking medication, don't lead to a total crisis, such as an infection.

Contrary to popular belief, healthy people often carry low levels of pathogens or disease-causing bacteria in their mouths.[48] But these pathogenic bacteria don't cause a problem because the mouth is protected by a strong defense of good commensal microbes.

Beneficial commensal organisms make chemicals that repel or destroy bad bacteria. They can even direct the immune system to a bad bug. It's as if they say to the immune cells, "Hey! There's the bad guy over there!"

Your good bacteria help to keep a strong mucosal barrier, thereby protecting you from the outside world. Commensal microbes prime, or teach, the immune system to tolerate "good bugs." As we discussed in Chapter 4, the immune system's default setting is inflammation and attack. Your commensal bacteria turn on T regulatory cells that teach acceptance and tolerance. With that knowledge, the immune system can spend its efforts seeking out and destroying bad bugs, not the good ones.[49] Your commensal microbes can even help make blood pressure–lowering chemicals that boost your cardiovascular health (more on this in Chapter 8).

As if that weren't enough, your commensal microbiota make nutrients and help you digest your food. Commensal bacteria make vitamin K, which helps your blood clot, builds healthy bones, and makes sure your blood flows smoothly through clean arteries. They also make biotin, a B vitamin that helps you make fuel from carbohydrates, fats, and proteins while giving you strong and beautiful hair, nails, and skin. Commensal bacteria ferment the food that you can't digest, making fatty acids (called short-chain fatty acids) that actually boost the health of your gut cells and can help to prevent colon cancer.[50] You can find a list of human commensal oral bacteria on page 157.

The Oral Mycobiome

While bacteria are the major players in the oral microbiome, fungi have a place in our mouths as well. Fungi make up a smaller percentage of the microbes in the mouth, with the average healthy mouth's mycobiome (or fungal biota) carrying 9 to 23 species. Candida is the most common fungal genus found in the mouth and *Candida albicans* is the most common species. Candida has been found on dental plaque.[51] Other fungal genera found in the mouth include Cladosporium, Aureobasidium, Saccharomyces, Aspergillus (or mold), Fusarium, and Cryptococcus.[52]

The Oral Virome

Viruses may trump the total bacteria count in the mouth by as much as 35 times![53] But most of these viruses in the oral virome (or viral biota) prey on bacteria, not humans. Bacteriophages are viruses that attack or even benefit bacteria. Therefore, wherever bacteria live (all over and in our bodies), bacteriophages live, too. Bacteriophages are the most numerous organisms on earth, and the diversity of bacteriophages closely aligns with the diversity of bacteria. Other viruses have been found in the oral cavity including herpes simplex virus (the virus that causes cold sores or genital herpes), varicella zoster virus (the virus that causes chickenpox or shingles), and human papilloma virus (the cause of warts on the skin or mucous membranes, including genital warts or cervical cancer).[54]

UNIQUE AS A SNOWFLAKE

Your personal oral microbiome is unique. This has been one of the challenges in understanding the microbiome, because we cannot easily define what is a normal microbiome and what is dysbiotic. Researchers are trying to characterize core microbiomes, or enterotypes, to help us address the tremendous variation in the bacteria that colonize us, which is totally normal and healthy. For example, in a study of the oral microbiota, the same 78 bacterial species were found in almost everyone (90 percent of participants). Yet 24 bacterial species were found in every single person (100 percent of participants).[55] Even though there is a lot of variety in the microbial communities in our mouths, there are common bugs that colonize most of us—hence a *core* microbiome.

Your oral microbiome is probably most similar to those of the people living in your home who eat a similar diet to you. You probably even share some oral microbes with your house pets! Laboratory testing , or at-home testing, of your oral microbiome is therefore helpful to monitor the makeup of your oral microbiome over time. We will talk about this in the "Testing" section of Chapter 9, Oral Microbiome Solutions.

THE ORIGINS OF YOUR MICROBIOME

So where do all of these microbes come from? Your mama. Seriously! You get your starter pack of bacteria, fungi, and viruses from your mother. And how we are born affects the oral microbiome and the gut microbiome. When a baby is slowly descending the birth canal, they get smeared with all of the vaginal microbes that colonize the mother. This is a major first inoculation. Lactobacillus bacteria are high in the vaginal microbiome, and babies born vaginally have high levels of this bug in their feces for their first few days of life. In fact, babies born vaginally end up with a gut microbiota that looks like their mom's, to the tune of 83 percent similar. And they have a rich, diverse collection of microbes, which is an indicator of microbial health.[56, 57]

With nearly one-third of babies in the United States being born by Cesarean section, not all babies get this starter pack, unfortunately. Babies born by C-section have a fecal microbiota that is only 42 percent similar to that of their mothers. Since C-section babies are not getting exposed to their mother's vaginal microbes, their microbiomes are composed of the bugs in their environment or the first things they touch or eat (like from mother's skin microbiota). The majority of babies that were born by C-section had high levels of the periodontal pathogen *Slackia exigua*, but babies born vaginally were free of this microbe. C-section babies also have less diversity in their oral microbiomes than babies born vaginally.[58, 59] Babies born by C-section are more likely to have asthma, allergies, and eczema, leading some experts to believe that the commensal bacteria from mother's vaginal microbiome is key in preventing these diseases.[60]

Breastfeeding also delivers a package of healthy microbes to the baby's mouth and gut. Breastmilk is high in probiotic bacteria *and* the prebiotics needed to feed them! Seeding the newborn gut with mother's bacteria promotes a healthy response to inflammation, helps introduce it to commensal bacteria, and jumpstarts the immune system. Breastmilk also contains immune-boosting proteins that can prevent the spread of pathogenic bacteria. Secretory IgA from mother's milk can destroy bacteria and protect the mucosal membranes. Delivering commensal bacteria, the prebiotics that feed them, and proteins that help to prevent dysbiosis means we have yet another thing to thank our moms for![61, 62]

PLAQUE AND BIOFILMS

All bacteria live in biofilm. A biofilm is a group of microorganisms that attach themselves to a surface and cover themselves with a protective shield (or slime). This mechanism helps microbes stay attached to a surface so that they don't get swept or washed away. The stuff that coats a biofilm is officially called "extracellular polymeric substance." It's made of polysaccharides, or a long chain of carbohydrates, which provide structure and can grab on to tougher minerals like magnesium and calcium to further strengthen the protective shield of the biofilm.

The first biofilm ever discovered was dental plaque! This was a tremendous realization to me, because we talk about microbial biofilms all the time when we talk about the gut microbiome. You might hear about treatments to break biofilms—these are used when trying to eliminate one or more pathogenic microbes.

Wherever there is microbial growth, it is pretty much guaranteed to be in biofilm. But biofilms don't just help protect bacteria and other bugs from being brushed away. A biofilm is like a little castle where microbes live. Inside the biofilm are little villages of bacteria, fungi, and other organisms. These "microcolonies" are typically separated by water channels.[63] For many years, scientists and doctors have been talking about bacteria as though they live in isolation. But just like humans, they live in communities with other microbes. They rarely live alone. Now it is widely accepted that microbes live in mixed ecological communities, not just a single microbe growing by itself in a petri dish.[64]

The microbes can also communicate with each other using chemical messages. They can live in harmony, but sometimes they compete with each other for control. The metabolic by-product of one bug can be a food source for another bug. Biofilms are a way that microbes can join together to protect themselves and survive treacherous conditions.[65]

Dental plaque was the first microbial biofilm ever discovered.

With their biofilm protection, microbes can evade the host immune system and dodge the lethal action of antibiotics. Biofilms make it easy for microbes to share genes that enhance their survival. The biofilm also appears to function as a unit, something that scientists call "quorum sensing." This means that the biofilm can turn on genes and release chemical messages to increase or decrease its size, to produce antibiotics, to release toxins, to cooperate with other microbes, and more. The bacterial biofilm therefore operates like an organism. It's pretty amazing that microbiota are able to do all of these things. Perhaps that's why they have so successfully colonized the far reaches of the planet![66, 67]

Every time you get a dental cleaning, your hygienist is scraping bacterial biofilms off of your teeth. Little villages of bacteria are being physically removed because their hard biofilm exterior makes it nearly impossible to get rid of them by brushing alone. Those are biofilms at work.

BACTERIA AND THE DIET

After you get your starter pack of microbes from your mother, other major contributors are the people around you, the environment you live in, and your diet. Bacteria are thrilled to inhabit the mouth, where there is a constant stream of yummy food. All of our bugs have evolved alongside us for millennia. They eat what we eat: the break-down products of protein, fiber, sugar, fats, and plants. Your microbiome really likes plant-based foods. A diet rich in fiber and vegetables but moderate in calories is practically guaranteed to benefit your microbiome, because fiber and vegetables are high in prebiotics. One of the most powerful ways to shift your microbiome is to eat more plant-based foods and fiber.

Prebiotics are the nondigestible carbohydrates from your diet that feed and grow beneficial microbes. This is basically the "bulk" from your diet. Since they aren't digestible, you can't use them for your own nutrition. Enter, your microbes. They ferment (or eat) prebiotics, which are usually nonstarch polysaccharides or oligosaccharides (long-chain or short-chain carbohydrates). When your microbes ferment prebiotics, they make short-chain fatty acids, which help prevent the overgrowth of bad bugs, boost the health of your mucosal lining, and can prevent cancer.[68] The more prebiotics you eat, the more you feed your good bugs, and the happier you and your bugs are. Examples of prebiotic foods are chicory root, Jerusalem artichoke, banana, and whole grain breakfast cereal.[69] You can also take prebiotics in the form of a nutritional supplement powder. Prebiotic supplements include galacto-oligosaccharides, inulin, and larch arabinogalactan.

HOW THE BUGS GOT THEIR NAMES

Before we talk about individual microbes, it will be helpful to do a quick primer on scientific names and taxonomy so you know what you're reading. A really brilliant scientist, Carl Linnaeus, figured out that we need ways to identify all of the cool plants and animals in the physical world. Each organism is taxonomically classified, meaning it has been organized and given a name in the bigger scheme of lifeforms on Earth. You probably remember this line-up from a biology class along the way:

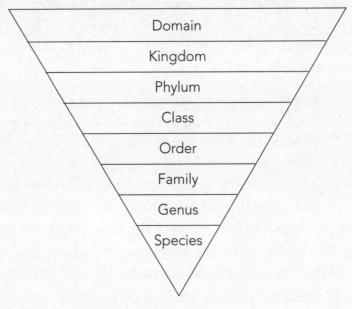

Figure 5.2: The taxonomic classification hierarchy.

Each species gets its own scientific name. It's usually two words, and they are both italicized. The first word is the genus and the second word is the species. The genus is often abbreviated. The chart below shows two examples: one for *Lactobacillus acidophilus*, a common probiotic bacteria, and one for *Escherichia coli* (*E. coli*) O157:H7, the bacterium that can cause food poisoning.

Taxonomic Classification of *E. coli* and *L. acidophilus*

DOMAIN	BACTERIA	BACTERIA
Kingdom	Bacteria	Bacteria
Phylum	Proteobacteria	Firmicutes
Class	Gamma-proteobacteria	Bacilli
Order	Enterobacteriales	Lactobacillales
Family	Enterobacteriaceae	Lactobacillaceae
Genus	Escherichia	Lactobacillus
Species	coli	acidophilus
Strain (subspecies, serotype, etc)	O157:H7	N/A
Species name	*Escherichia coli* O157:H7 or *E. coli* O157:H7	*Lactobacillus acidophilus*

Species name is very important as you learn about the microbiome. There can be many species within one genus. For instance, *Lactobacillus acidophilus* is in the Lactobacillus genus, but so are *Lactobacillus plantarum* and *Lactobacillus rhamnosus.*

I also want to emphasize the phylum (phyla, when plural). As you can tell from the taxonomic hierarchy, the phylum is a very high level of category, almost as high up on the hierarchy as kingdom. Certain phyla are very important in the human microbiome. As we continue, we will be talking about the Bacteroidetes and Firmicutes phyla. They happen to be the dominant players in the gut microbiome and the oral microbiome. Other important phyla in the oral microbiome are Proteobacteria, Actinobacteria, and Fusobacteria.[70]

As we discussed earlier, just because the gums, tongue, tonsils, saliva, and nose are all close to each other doesn't mean they have similar microbiomes! Take a look at the figure on page 65 to see how the different phyla are represented in the mouth and nose. Different microbial communities are seen on the gums, tongue, tonsils, and saliva. Firmicutes and Bacteroidetes phylum make up over half of the oral microbiome at all of those sites. Fusobacteria and Proteobacteria also are represented there, but in smaller portions. Actinobacteria is mostly on the sidelines in the mouth, but dominates the nose.

Phyla are the high-level "buckets" of bacteria in the microbiome. When we are talking about a genus or an individual species, we are taking a more detailed view of a microbe. Streptococcus species is one of the dominant players in the oral microbiome (Streptococcus is a genus and there are many individual species that fall within that genus). Streptococcus has a large representation in the saliva, gums, tongue, and tonsils. It is also present in the cheeks, roof of the mouth, and in dental plaque above and below the gumline (see the Summary of Human Commensal Oral Microbiota on page 157). When it comes to the oral microbiome, Streptococcus is a major part of the community!

Streptococcus species are the most abundant bacteria in the mouth.

In addition to Streptococcus, other common genera in the mouth are Fusobacterium (referring to the genus in this instance, not to be confused with the related, but much bigger, Fusobacteria phyla, above), Gemella, Neisseria, Rothia, and Veillonella. These groups of bacteria give us protection against infection, tune our immune systems, and help us keep a strong barrier against outside invaders.

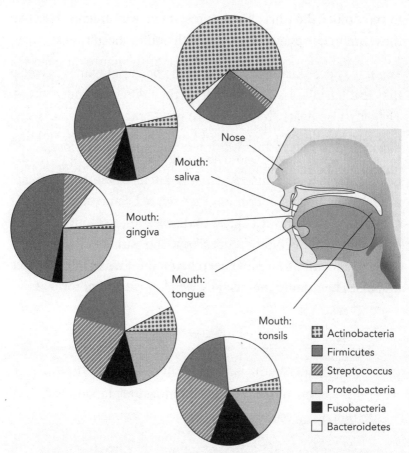

Figure 5.3: Bacterial composition of distinct ecological niches in the oral cavity and nose. Firmicutes phyla includes the genus Streptococcus. Bacteroidetes and Firmicutes make up over 50 percent of microbes in the mouth. Fusobacteria and Proteobacteria phyla are also represented, but less so. Actinobacteria dominates the nose, though it is also found in the mouth.

As I've mentioned, the oral microbiome includes 770 species with 20 billion microbes. It's impossible—and not very practical—to learn them all, so I have compiled a list of the more common microbes that are found in the human oral cavity from birth through adulthood (see page 157). The table also shows where the bugs live in the oral cavity and whether they colonize us when we are babies or only when we are adults. Try to remember the phyla Firmicutes and Bacteroidetes, because these are major players in the mouth and in the gut.

You have never heard of most of these bacterial names because they are harmless or beneficial, so they don't get much press. They are also nearly impossible to pronounce. But don't sweep them under the rug. These good bugs can save lives by holding up a biological defense and keeping bad bugs at bay. In the next chapter, we will discuss what happens when the beneficial microbes in the oral microbiome get out of balance and how that can lead to a downward spiral of disease in the mouth and the body. Later, we will talk more about the pathogenic microbial species, the ones that have been blamed for all of our diseases and ills. Their names are usually well known and notorious.

Takeaways

- Your commensal bacteria help protect you from infection and teach your immune system who is good and bad.

- Your microbiota are not loners; they live in complex biofilm communities. Plaque was the first biofilm ever discovered.

- Bacteria use biofilms to protect themselves, trade DNA, get resources, and evade the immune system and antibiotics.

- How you were born and if you were breastfed can significantly affect your microbiome.

- Over 40 percent of the oral microbiome is still unnamed and uncharacterized.

- Streptococcus species are the most abundant bacteria in the oral cavity.

- Bacteroidetes and Firmicutes are the dominant phyla in the oral microbiome and in the gut microbiome.

CHAPTER 6

DYSBIOSIS OF THE ORAL MICROBIOME

"Every tooth in a man's head is more valuable than a diamond."

—Miguel de Cervantes, author of *Don Quixote*

What do cavities, gingivitis, periodontal disease, root canals, and bad breath all have in common? They are *all* examples of dysbiosis of the microbiota in our mouths. It appears that our oral microbiome packs a punch! So, let's not underestimate the bugs that live in and on us. An unhappy oral microbiome can make us unhappy on an everyday basis. In this chapter, we will talk about how imbalanced oral bugs can lead to problems right there in the mouth. In later chapters, we will see how that dysbiosis can spiral out of control and even harm our joints, gut, and cardiovascular systems.

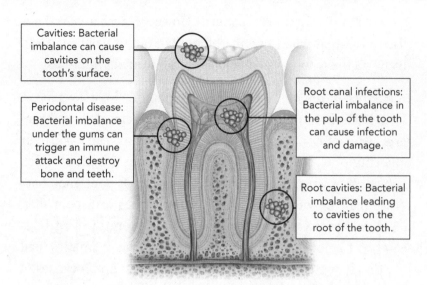

Figure 6.1: Dysbiosis of the oral microbiota can cause cavities, root canal infections, and periodontal disease. Dysbiotic microbiota affect the crowns of the teeth (cavities), the pulp of the tooth (root canal infections), the roots of the teeth (root cavities), and the gums, periodontal ligament, and bone (periodontal disease).

In Chapter 1 we compared the microbiome to a rich, healthy rainforest. We spelled out what that environment looks like in Chapter 3. And in the previous chapter, we learned that the microbes living in our mouths live in sophisticated colonies (or biofilms) that help them survive harsh conditions and sequester resources. Bacteroidetes and Firmicutes are two dominant phyla in the healthy mouth. And Streptococcus species are a major player in the oral microbiome. All of our oral microbes co-exist within us peacefully, often helping us.

But what happens if this harmonious microbial balance in the mouth is disturbed? The result is dysbiosis. As you learned in Chapter 2, dysbiosis is an imbalance in the normal microbial make-up. Each person has a unique microbial pattern, so there is no definitive "normal" microbial balance. Likewise, there is no definitive dysbiosis pattern. However, researchers have discovered that when the microbiota fall out of balance, it can throw off the whole system and cause unwanted symptoms.

Imbalance in the microbiome can happen in a lot of scenarios. Good bacteria can overgrow and cause problems. "Shady" bacteria, who often hang out in the background, can take their opportunity to overgrow. You can get a true infection, which throws all of your microbiota out of whack. Or your good bacteria might be weak, either due to antibiotics or a poor diet, and they leave you open to infection or overgrowth of bugs who don't belong there. Oral dysbiosis can cause cavities, bad breath, gingivitis, and periodontal disease. Common causes of dysbiosis include:[71, 72]

- Antibiotics

- Infection

- Low levels of good bacteria

- Low fiber/poor diet

- Medications

- Poor saliva flow (dry mouth)

- Sugar

- Weakened immune system

THE MICROBIAL ECOLOGY
OF CAVITIES

Cavities are the break-down of teeth due to acids made by bacteria. Cavities are little holes in the hard surface of the tooth and can affect the crown or the root. When cavities reach the pulp of the teeth, which houses nerves and blood supply, a root canal may be needed.

One in three Americans has untreated tooth decay and the vast majority have some form of gum disease.[73] Cavities cause toothache, tooth sensitivity, holes or pits in teeth, pain when eating or drinking, and stains on the surface of the tooth.

Periodontal disease and cavities are the most common oral diseases of humankind.[74]

Until recently, a single bacterium was thought to cause cavities: the infamous *Streptococcus mutans* (or *S. mutans*, for short). However, scientific discoveries have taught us that it is not *one single bug* causing the problem, but instead an overall shift in the oral microecology that sets the stage for cavities.

In a healthy mouth, Streptococcus and Lactobacilli bacteria are the major players. These normal, harmless forms of Streptococcus make up 95 percent of dental plaque: *Streptococcus sanguinis*, *Streptococcus oralis*, and *Streptococcus mitis*. (Remember, dental plaque is bacteria on the teeth.) Meanwhile, the "bad bug" *S. mutans* is only found in 2 percent of the bacterial biofilms in a healthy mouth.[75] In this scenario, notice that the good bugs are keeping the bad bug at bay. *S. mutans* is present, but harmless.

However, if you aren't keeping up with your dental hygiene, if you're eating sugar, and if your saliva isn't flowing well, it increases acid in your mouth, which sets off a chain of events that disrupts the bacteria that live on your teeth and causes cavities. As the acid in the

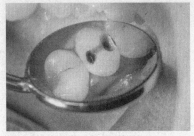

A disruption of the bacteria that live on your teeth can lead to dental cavities.

mouth increases, it primes the environment for making cavities. The good bugs start to die off. *S. mutans* starts to feel more comfortable and spreads its wings. It can then take over and bring some friends. *Streptococcus sobrinus*, Bifidobacteria, Candida (yeast), Actinomyces, and Lactobacillus start to move in and take over, too, crowding out the healthy bacteria of the past.[76] Candida is high in cavity dysbiosis, and *S. mutans* and Candida seem to cooperate and help each other to create cavities.[77] As these new bugs take over, they promote a whole new microbiotic regime that allows only a few certain bugs to thrive and kills off the masses of good bugs that were protective. Over time, the community of microbes changes and matures, and does more damage to the tooth. Cavities get worse. The bacteria that live in the cavity are very different from the bacteria living elsewhere in the healthy mouth; this community is even under study by scientists because cavities have a microbiome of their own.[78] See the chart on page 158 for a list of microbes involved in cavities, gingivitis, periodontal disease, and more.

This is a very important concept and one that I hope you will remember when you walk away from this book. It is not a single, solitary bug that is wreaking total havoc. It is usually the microecology that has been disturbed and is therefore leaving you (the host) vulnerable to disease. Some healthcare practitioners call the microecology the "terrain": If the host's terrain is unhealthy or damaged, then a single pathogen can cause major trouble. But if the terrain is healthy, has lots of diverse microbiota who are living in harmony with you, and has a strong barrier, then you are unlikely to have any trouble—even though bad bugs may be hanging around. They just can't get their foot in the door to cause any real problems because the good bugs never give them an opportunity.

Streptococcus mutans and *Streptococcus sobrinus* are usually detected in the oral microbiome when someone has cavities. However, in one research study of teenagers who had cavities, 15 to 30 percent had no *S. mutans*. That's because other acid-producing oral bacteria can also cause cavities, not just *S. mutans*. These include Lactobacilli, Bifidobacteria, and non-mutans Streptococci and Actinomyces species.[79] For this reason, dietary changes like cutting out sugar and reducing acid can be among the most powerful ways to control your oral microbiome (check out Chapter 9 for more details).

A three-year-old boy, Grayson, had terrible cavities. His mother took him to Dr. Donna Ruiz, desperately seeking alternatives. Grayson's dentist was recommending that he have a "pulpectomy" under general anesthesia. A pulpectomy is a root canal therapy that removes all of the tissue inside the tooth. It's usually recommended when infection has worked its way throughout the pulp and into the root canal system.

At age two, Grayson already had many cavities. Almost every tooth on the top half of his mouth had extensive tooth decay. His parents had food sensitivities so Grayson was already on a gluten-free, sugar-free, dairy-free, and nut-free diet. His mother also said Grayson had some behavioral issues and threw tantrums easily, even with normal challenges. Grayson had nutritional issues since birth and had colic, thrush, and diaper rash while a baby.

Dr. Ruiz did testing and designed a comprehensive treatment to heal Grayson's mouth. She tried to shift Grayson's oral microbiome using a probiotic toothpaste (PerioBiotic, by Designs for Health), the oral bacteria *Streptococcus salivarius* (ProbioMax DDS from Xymogen), and a children's chewable probiotic (UltraFlora Chew by Metagenics). She had him do a tea tree solution oral rinse to lower bacteria in the mouth. Dr. Ruiz tested and restored some of his nutrients like vitamin D and B vitamins. She built up his immune system and gave him homeopathic medications to help strengthen his teeth and bones. She recommended that Grayson use xylitol as a sweetener and eat more plums since those could inhibit *S. mutans*, the bacteria commonly present in cavities.

The treatment totally arrested Grayson's tooth decay. It fixed his bad teeth. He didn't have to get the pulpectomy. Even his behavioral issues improved. Grayson was doing so much better that he no longer needed treatment. When he came back for treatment one year later, it wasn't for cavities. It was because his behavioral issues were cropping up again.

SUGAR IS THE PITS

If you are like me, you've been told that sugar is bad for your teeth a million times. But do you know why? When you eat sugar, you are feeding bacteria in your mouth. Bacteria break down sugar and carbohydrates and produce acids. Acid helps set the stage for cavities. As things get more acidic in the mouth, it encourages even more acid-loving bacteria to climb on board.[80] What do they do? Make more acid!

In Chapter 3, we discussed how incredibly hard and tough teeth are, but they are no match for a high-acid environment and a bunch of acid-producing bacteria. When high levels of acid damage the enamel (the protective, hard layer on the teeth), the tooth breaks down and is vulnerable to further attack from bacteria. Sugary and acidic soft drinks are also an archnemesis of healthy teeth.[81] Sugar destroys teeth, but with the help of oral bacteria.

The oral microbiota is stable and in harmony with the host, unless disturbed by medication, disease, low pH, or significant changes in diet.[82]

GINGIVITIS AND PERIODONTAL DISEASE

One out of two people in the United States has a history of gingivitis. Its more advanced form, periodontitis, affects nearly 50 percent of people over the age of 30.[83] Periodontal disease, which includes gingivitis and periodontitis, is caused by dysbiosis of the oral microbiome and the immune system's reaction to it.

However, if bacterial biofilms (a.k.a. plaque) under the gumline grow out of control, the immune system launches chemical and biological warfare against the microbes that have gotten out of control. It is similar to lighting a fire in the gums. It's all well and good if this chemical and biological fire effectively kills the unwanted bacteria. But if it doesn't work, what do you think is the result? Periodontitis. Sadly, the unchecked inflammation destroys gums, eats away at bone, strips the ligaments that hold the teeth in place, and eventually the tooth loosens and falls out. As the bone and gums that used to surround and hold the tooth snugly break down, something called a "periodontal pocket" opens up next to the tooth, which fills with even *more* bacterial biofilms. Bad news.

Periodontal disease doesn't just harm the mouth—it can affect the whole body. Having periodontitis increases your risk of whole-body diseases such as atherosclerosis (hardening of the arteries), diabetes (blood sugar dysregulation), and cancer. We will talk more about the mind-blowing associations between periodontal disease and a long list of other systemic diseases in Chapter 8.

Periodontal disease is an umbrella term that includes gingivitis and mild, moderate, and severe periodontitis.[84] The term comes from the word "periodontium," which refers to the gums (or gingivae), ligaments, and bone that hug and hold each tooth securely in the mouth. If your gums are red, irritated, or bleeding, that is a sign of gingivitis, an early form of periodontal disease that causes swollen, puffy, receding, sometimes tender gums. It means that your immune system is not happy and is trying to attack your oral microbiota. If gingivitis goes untreated, it can worsen to periodontitis, which damages the gums, bone, and even causes tooth loss, as described previously.

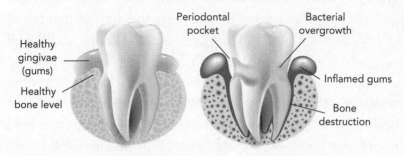

Healthy Tooth/Gum   Diseased Tooth/Gum

Healthy gingivae (gums)

Healthy bone level

Periodontal pocket

Bacterial overgrowth

Inflamed gums

Bone destruction

Figure 6.2: Periodontal disease compared to healthy gums. The body launches an immune attack on overgrown bacterial communities, which destroys gum and bone tissue. The resulting "pocket" fills with more bacteria, worsening the inflammation and further damaging the gums and bone, and can eventually lead to tooth loss.

In the 1600s, "teeth" was listed as a leading cause of death by the London (England) Bills of Mortality. Dental abscess was still a leading cause of death even 200 years ago.[85]

The great news about gingivitis: It is easy to treat! Regular flossing and brushing and dental cleanings can help reduce the bacterial overgrowth on the teeth, turn off the immune system attack, and heal and soothe the gums. If you have periodontal disease, see a dentist and a periodontist you trust for further treatment. Cavities, gingivitis, and periodontal disease can all be traced back to disturbances in your oral microbiome, so treatments to rebalance the microbiome can turn around these conditions. Avoid sugar and packaged foods (a.k.a. refined carbohydrates) like the plague, eat more vegetables and fiber, use chewable probiotics or probiotic toothpaste, take high doses of oral probiotics (50 million CFU/day or more), and review the additional Oral Microbiome Solutions in Chapter 9 to put a cap on bacterial overgrowth in the mouth.

BAD BREATH

Everyone complains of bad breath once in a while. But persistent bad breath is a whole other issue. Although it isn't dangerous, it is a sign of oral disease or imbalance. Bad breath is commonly caused by oral bacterial action on food particles. When a person slacks off on brushing and flossing and visiting the dentist, microbes build up on the teeth and tongue. These bacteria are thrilled to inhabit the mouth, where there is a constant stream of yummy food. But when our oral microbes eat, they make waste products, including gases. Certain bacterial species make characteristic by-products that stink. If those bugs overgrow in the mouth, it can cause bad breath. Gingivitis and periodontal disease are characterized by microbial overgrowth and inflammation and can also cause varying degrees of bad breath.[86]

Remember in Chapter 3 when we talked about how a regular flow of saliva keeps the mouth healthy? Saliva cleanses the mouth and keeps the microbiota in check. If you have a dry mouth, it can lead to dysbiosis in the mouth and bad breath. Revisit your dental hygiene (brushing, flossing, and dental cleanings) to get a handle on microbial dysbiosis and bad breath. Remember to brush your tongue, which can hold leftover food particles and lots of microbiota.

The most obvious cause of bad breath is right there in the mouth. However, if you have good oral health, then bad breath might be coming from dysbiosis or disease in the sinuses, throat, lungs, or even the gastrointestinal tract. Bad breath is occasionally a symptom of a systemic disease that might be more serious.[87]

TOXIC BY-PRODUCTS OF BAD BACTERIA

Just like us, bacteria eat and make waste products. As we mentioned earlier in this chapter, bacteria can make harmful levels of acid in the mouth, causing cavities. Plaque bacteria can make chemicals like hydrogen sulfide, ammonia, enzymes, and proteins that trigger the inflammatory response. In moderation, the inflammatory response to these toxic by-products is effective. If the inflammatory response spirals out of control, it is dangerous and can cause periodontal disease or worse.[88]

Some bacterial by-products are extremely poisonous for us. Lipopolysaccharide (LPS) is a particularly toxic component of a gram-negative bacteria's cell wall. It is infamous for triggering serious inflammation in the host and can even cause life-threatening conditions from bacterial infections. When it binds to immune cells, they get vicious, unleashing biological warfare to eliminate the threat. LPS gets such a huge rise from the immune system that researchers even use LPS in experimental models of inflammation.

Take Control of Your Oral Microbiome

Dysbiosis of the mouth is a serious affair, but it can be treated. Regular, long-term dental care can change your oral microbiota and your chances of cavities, gum disease, and bad breath.[89] Your diet, when low in sugar and refined carbohydrates, can encourage a healthier microbiome. Probiotics can reduce *S. mutans* and reduce cavities.[90] You can review these and other oral microbiome solutions that will help you get in the driver's seat, take control of your oral microbiome, and reduce the risk of oral diseases in Chapter 9.

ORAL-SYSTEMIC CONNECTION

If you are swallowing 140 billion bacterial cells every day, what would this mean for the mouth's downstream counterpart, the gastrointestinal tract? Dysbiosis in the mouth could take a ride on the waterslide and dive into the stomach, small intestine, or large intestine.

The mouth and the gut are kissing cousins with a shared architecture, immune network, and mucosal barrier. Every time you swallow, you are seeding your gastrointestinal tract with the bacteria, fungi, and viruses from your mouth—140 billion per day, to be exact. This means that in terms of the gut microbiome alone, the mouth is a major contributor to what is happening in the gut. In fact, researchers have shown that there is a 45 percent overlap in the microbes from the mouth and the gut, proving how closely related these two microbiomes are. There is more bacterial diversity in the gut and oral microbiomes than anywhere else in the body. Disease in the mouth can therefore be mirrored in the gut, and I would venture to say that you must have a healthy oral microbiome in order to have a healthy gut microbiome.

But that isn't all. Bacterial dysbiosis in the mouth can end up outside of the GI tract, too. Remember that you will find blood vessels and nerves at the center of each tooth, called the pulp. Suffice it to say that *each and every tooth has access to the bloodstream.* So, if there is dysbiosis of bacteria on the teeth, under the gums, inside the teeth, or anywhere in the mouth, it can effectively reach the bloodstream and use it to travel to far-off sites in the body. In the case of a root canal infection, which is an infection or dysbiosis of the pulp of the tooth, those bacteria could hitch a ride on the blood superhighway and eventually land in a knee joint or even in the heart. Likewise, the inflammation from gingivitis and periodontal disease can slide right into the bloodstream, delivering toxic chemicals to other parts of the body.

> *Some tortures are physical*
> *And some are mental,*
> *But the one that is both*
> *Is dental.*
> —Ogden Nash, American humorist

The oral cavity is intimately linked to systemic circulation. This is a fascinating topic called the oral-systemic connection that thrills experts and consumers alike and is the topic of the next chapters. So, read on for something that will blow your mind: how the mouth can influence total-body health.

COMMENSAL BACTERIA
OR PATHOGEN?

Certain periodontal pathogens are uniquely able to create disease, evade the immune system defenses, penetrate the tissues, and activate inflammation and tissue destruction.[91] Three species of bacteria, referred to as the red complex, are believed to be involved in gum disease: *Porphyromonas gingivalis, Tannerella forsythia, and Treponema denticola. Porphyromonas gingivalis* in particular has been historically believed to be the cause of periodontal disease because it activates inflammation and bone loss.[92] We will be talking about *P. gingivalis* a lot in Chapter 8, especially when we talk about periodontal pathogens that have been found in heart disease plaques and rheumatoid arthritis joints. Candida and oral viruses have also been implicated in periodontal dysbiosis.[93]

There is a fine line between commensal organisms and pathogens in the oral microbiome. Healthy individuals from the Human Microbiome Project were found to commonly carry oral pathogens, albeit at low levels. In the mouths of many of the study subjects, scientists found pathogenic organisms that can cause periodontal and root canal infections, cavities, periodontitis, pneumonia, strep throat, scarlet fever, meningitis, blood infections, and ear and sinus infections. Yet all of these people were completely healthy. The high prevalence of these microbes in healthy people led scientists to conclude that they were actually commensal organisms and would be involved in disease only when there was oral dysbiosis.[94]

For a full list of microbes, see "Oral Microbes Involved in Disease" on page 158.

Porphyromonas gingivalis and *Streptococcus mutans* are present when there is dysbiosis and disease in the mouth. But *P. gingivalis* can also be a normal, commensal bacteria because it is present in the oral microbiomes of people who are perfectly healthy.[95] Likewise, *S. mutans*, the infamous microbial cause of cavities, isn't always present in people with cavities.[96] Even in populations who have excellent oral hygiene care, still 1 in 5 people gets cavities.

Obviously, *S. mutans* isn't always the single cause of cavities and *P. gingivalis* isn't the single cause of gum disease. There is a variety of bacteria involved in periodontal disease and cavities. Periodontal disease is suggestive of a bigger problem: a dysbiosis of the oral microbiota and an aberrant immune response to them. It is an overall shift in the microbial ecology in the mouth that allows certain microbes to rise to power and do damage. A healthy oral microbiome prevents this from happening.

An interview with functional dentist Dr. Mary Ellen Chalmers taught me that doing everything "right" to prevent cavities doesn't work for everyone. There are people who do everything they should do, like eating a healthy diet, brushing, flossing, and seeing the dentist regularly, but they still get cavities. There are people who eat a lot of sugar and simple carbs, don't brush regularly, and don't floss, and they *don't* get cavities! Dentists can't always explain this. Oral disease doesn't just depend on your oral hygiene and your oral microbiome. An interplay of genetics, environment, microbes, immune system, and maybe even blind luck determine whether you are prone to cavities or not (see more about this in Chapter 10).

Takeaways

- Cavities, gingivitis, periodontal disease, and bad breath are examples of oral dysbiosis.

- Sugar and packaged foods (those containing refined carbohydrates) promote dysbiosis of the oral microbiome and oral diseases.

- It is no longer believed that one microbe single-handedly causes disease; instead, a shift in the microbial ecology allows harmful bacteria to rise to power.

- Periodontal disease is a chronic inflammatory disease caused by microbial imbalance and excessive immune reactions.

- Oral dysbiosis may arise when various interrelated factors are not kept in balance: diet, salivary flow, pH environment, immune defenses, and microbial balance.

CHAPTER 7

KISSING COUSINS: THE GUT AND THE MOUTH

"The oral cavity serves as a window into the intestinal tract."

—M. J. Docktor et al.[97]

If you have been waiting to read about the magnificent microbiome of the gut, here is your opportunity! The gut microbiome is a heavyweight compared to the oral microbiome. But the mouth and the gut have so many similarities, there is no way to talk about them except as intimately interrelated—as kissing cousins. In Chapters 3, 4, and 5 we talked about the mucosal membrane, the immune system, and the complex communities of microbes that live in our mouths, respectively. In this chapter we can see how the prime location of the mouth can directly influence the gut microbiome. We may be able to trace the origins of diseases in the gut back to the mouth. In this way, the oral cavity is linked not only with the entire GI tract but also with the rest of the body.

THE ALMIGHTY GUT

The gastrointestinal tract has been in the spotlight for centuries. Even Hippocrates thought the gut was vital to health when he said, "All disease begins in the gut." Indeed, many clinicians who treat the root causes of disease, not just the symptoms, often restore health to the gut first because it can influence health of the immune system, liver, joints, skin, brain, and more. The gastrointestinal tract is a series of hollow organs joined together in a long twisting tube that is nearly 30 feet long from mouth to anus, and whose surface area covers the space of a studio apartment. It includes the mouth, pharynx, esophagus, stomach, small intestines, large intestines, and rectum. The GI tract is the machinery that helps us eat, drink, digest food, absorb nutrients, and get rid of waste. It does all of those things while still acting as a physical barrier against outside invaders and policing the forefront of the immune battlefield to keep bad stuff out of the systemic circulation (the bloodstream), where it doesn't belong.

Seventy percent of your immune system lives in your gut. It monitors all of the foreign molecules passing through and will launch a fierce attack at the first hint of a malicious invader.

The gut walks a tightrope between inflammation and peaceful harmony. But generally, the gut tries to keep things calm, harmonious, and in good working order. The immune system, which is so important in the gut, permeates the mouth in just the same way.

Hearkening back to earlier chapters, the landmark collaboration to characterize the human microbiome, the Human Microbiome Project funded by the National Institutes of Health, taught us that the human gut harbors *100 trillion bacteria* that influence nutrition, immune function, metabolism, obesity, mood, cancer initiation, and susceptibility to infection. The gut also has its own nervous system, the enteric nervous system, which has been called the "second brain." There are 200 to 600 million neurons in the gut, which use more than 30 neurotransmitters (brain chemicals). Additionally, 95 percent of the body's good mood chemical, serotonin, is found in the gut.[98]

Compared to the gut's 100 trillion bacteria, its kissing cousin, the mouth, is estimated to have only 20 billion microbes. The vast majority of our microbial inhabitants live in the gastrointestinal tract and that is why there has been, with good reason, a flurry of scientific research and consumer books about the gut microbiome. As discussed in Chapter 3, dysbiosis of the gut microbiome seems to be involved in a range of intestinal illnesses such as Crohn's disease, ulcerative colitis, celiac disease, *Clostridium difficile*–associated diarrhea, and much more. Because the gut is so critical to overall health, evaluating and restoring gut function is a foundational clinical strategy in integrative and functional medicine. If you are looking for superior medical help with chronic illness, see Chapter 9, to find a functional medical practitioner in your area.

Gut dysbiosis symptoms and conditions include:

- Abdominal pain

- Asthma

- Autoimmune disease

- Bloating

- Constipation

- Diarrhea

- Eczema

- Gas

- Heartburn

- Inflammatory bowel disease

- Intestinal permeability (leaky gut)

- Irritable bowel syndrome

- Joint pain due to an infection in the joint

- Overweight or obesity

- Small intestinal bacterial overgrowth (SIBO)

- Ulcer

- Vomiting

SIMILARITIES BETWEEN THE GUT AND THE MOUTH

Just by virtue of anatomy, the mouth is unavoidably hitched to the gut. The mouth and the gut share an epithelial lining that acts as a permeable physical barrier, responsible for keeping bad stuff out and letting good stuff in (discussed in Chapter 3). The mucosal membranes in the mouth and the gut are populated with a formidable immune defense, including cells that guard and police, those that fingerprint and book enemies at the headquarters, and "soldier" cells that replicate themselves, hunt down, and destroy enemies (covered in Chapter 4).

The mouth and the gut are loaded with microbes that mostly contribute to healthy metabolism, physiology, and immunology, but at times contribute to disease. In both the gut and the mouth, a healthy person carries around pathogens that give them no problem, as long as they have a strong, diverse microbiome. But dysbiosis of the oral or gut microbiome can open the window for a bad bug rising to power. Dysbiosis, together with immune reactions, can cause disease in the mouth and the gut. The foods we eat dramatically influence the microbes in our mouths and in our guts. And as mentioned in Chapter 5, how we are born (vaginal or C-section) and how we are nursed can either give us a healthy, diverse microbiome or a weak, puny microbiome in both places.

The mouth and gut are just two stops on the same bus line. *Of course* they are connected in terms of their microbes, their immune responses, and their diseases! And I hesitate to say problems in the mouth that are mirrored in the gut are "systemic diseases," meaning diseases that affect the entire body, because the mouth is simply upstream of the gut. It's the same tube, just farther down.

So many things you learn in this book about the oral microbiome can also be used to understand the gut microbiome (and the gut). And since these kissing cousins are so similar, after reading this book you can consider yourself knowledgeable not only about the mouth, but about the gut as well.

LOCATION IS EVERYTHING

You've heard me say it before and you'll hear me say it again. The mouth is at the headwaters of the gastrointestinal tract, and the mouth is where the immune system first encounters the outside world. In its infinite wisdom, it tags suspicious outsiders with the help of the immune protein called sIgA (page 43) and sends communications to the gut immune system to beware of and prepare for them. The microbial communities living in the mouth flow downstream by way of saliva to the tune of 140 billion bacteria per day![99, 100, 101] The mouth is therefore "seeding" the rest of the gastrointestinal tract with microbes on a daily basis.

It is no surprise, then, that human microbiome scientists have found a whopping 45 percent overlap between the oral and colonic microbiota. Nearly 50 percent of the microbiomes in the oral cavity and the gut are the same. Bacteroidetes and Firmicutes phyla bacteria are dominant in both the oral and gut microbiomes. As I mentioned previously, one reason I have come to love the oral microbiome is that it strongly influences the composition of the gut microbiome.[102]

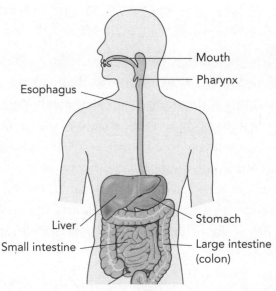

Figure 7.1: The human digestive tract includes the mouth, pharynx, esophagus, stomach, small intestine, large intestine, and anus. Since the mouth is at the headwaters of the gastrointestinal tract, it has an influence on everything downstream.

The constant flowing of saliva, chewing of food, and brushing of teeth removes bacteria from the oral cavity and pushes them downstream, toward the GI tract.[103] This is great if there is a healthy, rich oral microbial ecology in the mouth. But if there is dysbiosis or pathogenic bacteria in the mouth, it can provide a continual source of problematic microbes to the gut. This could result in chronic, recurrent dysbiosis in the stomach, small intestine, or colon that are resistant to the usual treatments.

There are two things in life that a sage must preserve at every sacrifice, the coats of his stomach and the enamel of his teeth. Some evils admit of consolations, but there are no comforters for dyspepsia and the toothache.
—Henry Lytton Bulwer, British politician, diplomat, and writer

HELICOBACTER PYLORI

Helicobacter pylori may be a perfect example of an unwelcome guest. *H. pylori* is a type of bacteria that can burrow into the epithelial lining of the stomach and damage the cells there. This exposes the underlying stomach tissues to very high acid levels, which makes matters worse and can even create sores called ulcers. Robin Warren and Barry Marshall were awarded the Nobel prize in 2005 for discovering that *H. pylori* could cause stomach ulcers, gastritis (inflammation of the stomach lining causing pain, nausea, vomiting, or a sense of fullness), and gastric cancer.

Helicobacter pylori has been evolving with us for well over 50,000 years.[104] In recent years, some researchers have suggested that *H. pylori* may not be a bad guy all the time. Many people have *H. pylori* and don't have any symptoms and never will. Since 50 percent of people have *H. pylori* and most have no symptoms, they say it may be a commensal organism and that it might even protect against developing certain allergies, esophageal cancer, heartburn, and obesity.[105, 106] This is often the confusion around microbes. They can be bad in certain situations and good in others. Labeling a microbe as "good" or "bad" is not cut and dry. It often depends on the other microbes in the mix and the person's immune system and environment.

I was surprised and fascinated to find out that *H. pylori* lives in dental plaques in the mouth! Researchers have discovered that when someone has a stomach infection with *H. pylori*, there's a good chance that it's living on their teeth as well. It seems that *H. pylori* living on the teeth can be a continuous source of *H. pylori* to the stomach, making it hard to get rid of even with all the appropriate treatments. In one study of people with stomach ulcers, those who had regular dental cleanings were able to get rid of *H. pylori* infection more effectively. For their counterparts who didn't get a dental cleaning to remove plaque, nearly 85 percent had a relapse of the *H. pylori* infection.[107, 108]

The moral of the story here is that if you have chronic upper GI symptoms, you and your doctor might want to review your oral health. Bacteria living on our teeth can take the "waterslide" down the esophagus and dive right into the stomach, small intestine, or large intestine.

INFLAMMATORY BOWEL DISEASE

There is some interesting overlap between bowel diseases and oral diseases, too. Inflammatory bowel diseases (IBD) such as Crohn's disease and ulcerative colitis affect approximately 250 out of every 100,000 Americans.[109, 110] These conditions are characterized by rampant, uncontrolled inflammation that leads to gastrointestinal tissue injury. People with IBD may have abdominal pain, diarrhea, rectal bleeding, fever, weight loss, and even malnutrition and vitamin deficiencies. The causes are yet unknown, but an over-the-top immune response to gut microbiota and damage to the intestinal barrier are central features of these diseases.[111, 112] Sound familiar?

Patients with IBD often have inflammation of the oral mucosa, too. Up to 80 percent of patients with Crohn's disease have symptoms of oral disease. In children who were newly diagnosed with Crohn's disease, 42 percent had oral symptoms. Inflammation in the mouth may be mild or severe, and it may begin *years* before any sign of inflammatory bowel disease begins.[113] This makes you wonder if the signs of illness show up first in the mouth.

People with inflammatory bowel disease often have lost some of the healthy diversity and richness of their intestinal micro-biome. One study found that in Crohn's disease, changes to the oral microbiota paralleled the changes in the intestinal microbiota. Both microbiomes were decreased and less diverse. They were both missing bacteria from the Fusobacteria and Firmicutes phyla.[114]

The First Time I Realized You Could Fix the Gut by Fixing the Mouth

When I worked at Metametrix Clinical Laboratory, I often reviewed lab results with a nutrition prac-titioner who grew to be a friend. In addition to running tests on her patients, "Jan" also ran tests on herself because she was trying to resolve some stubborn gut symptoms. Jan had indigestion, stomach pain, bloating, and loose stools even though she had an extraordinarily healthy diet for many years and took supplements to keep her gut healthy and improve digestion. Jan ran a urinary organic acids test, which measures by-products of bacteria that live in the small intestine. Jan's test showed very high levels of these bacterial metabolites, so we knew that she had high amounts of bacterial overgrowth in her small intestine. Her test results matched her chronic gut symptoms. Jan treated herself with antimicrobial herbs, digestive enzymes, and made changes to her diet to try to cure herself of bacterial dysbiosis, but to no avail. She ran a few tests on herself over the course of two years and every time, her gut showed rampant bacterial overgrowth, resistant to any and all treatments. Since her mother had not breastfed her, we wondered if her stubborn dysbiosis had begun when she was a baby and perhaps was unchangeable. Finally, one day Jan called in to discuss another set of her test results, like we had every other time. But this time the results looked completely normal. Jan had resolved her bacterial dysbiosis for the first time in years! I was stunned and of course asked her, "What did you do?!" Jan told me that she had been to the periodontist to resolve some mouth issues she was having. Ever since, her gut symptoms seemed to be getting better, and eventually subsided. By improving her oral health, Jan had resolved her chronic GI symptoms and normalized her test results. Jan's case stuck with me forever because it showed me that the mouth plays an important role in gut health.

Patients with IBD are more likely to have periodontal disease and inflamed, loose, bleeding gums. They are also more likely to have worse dysbiosis under the gumline than people who only have periodontal disease without bowel disease.[115]

It is hard to determine which one comes first: inflammatory bowel disease or periodontal disease. We don't know, and it may be a long time before we do, but there are striking similarities between the two conditions, including dysbiosis of the microbiota, damage to the mucosal membranes, and altered immune responses. In the meantime, experts suggest simultaneously treating the inflammation in the mouth *and* in the gut as a way to battle the combined challenge of oral disease and gastrointestinal disease.[116] See Oral Microbiome Solutions (Chapter 9) for ideas on how to lower inflammation in the mouth, improve the oral microbiome, and eat foods that promote a healthier mouth and gut. If you struggle with IBD and periodontal disease, I strongly encourage you to find a functional medicine practitioner or a licensed naturopathic doctor to help you get a handle on both of these conditions and get your health back on track. Recommendations for finding a qualified practitioner are also located in Chapter 9.

MY JOURNEY TO THE MOUTH BEGAN WITH POOP

With an interest in natural medicine and a history studying medicinal plants in the rainforests of Panama, I started my career in natural product drug discovery at a start-up company at the University of Georgia. Shortly thereafter, my friend and labmate, Dr. Eve Bralley, suggested I apply for a job at her family company, Metametrix Clinical Laboratory. They sold lab tests to integrative doctors that helped figure out if a patient had healthy levels of vitamins, minerals, and hormones; whether they had food allergies; and more.

Not long after I started the job, Metametrix launched a test that had never been done by any other clinical laboratory up to that point. It was a stool test that used DNA technology to detect bacteria and fungi in the gut. There were many stool tests on the market, but none that used this state-of-the-art technology. We were applying something brand new and it took the market by storm. My job was to research, write, and teach about microbes in the gut and help doctors use our stool tests to get their patients well again.

Years later, I started my own medical communications business, and I was commissioned by Klaire Labs to write an article on the oral microbiome with Dr. Stephen Olmstead. You can imagine my delight! The topic of microbiology was near and dear to my heart after reviewing thousands of poop tests. The article was right up my alley and I loved writing it.

My dear friend and teacher Dr. Kara Fitzgerald, whom I knew from Metametrix, asked me to be a guest on her functional medicine podcast to discuss what I had learned about the oral microbiome while writing the paper. Our interview was a huge hit and she had a record number of viewers! For some reason, doctors and dentists loved the topic as much as we did.

A number of people sought me out after the podcast interview, including Dr. Mark Burhenne, a prominent dentist with a large online following. I did an interview with him and I continued to write blogs and articles on the topic. Finally, Ulysses Press contacted me. They felt that the market was ready for an oral microbiome book and the online articles and interviews led them straight to me. I was thrilled to be offered the opportunity.

Takeaways

- The gut microbiome is of major interest because gut health powerfully affects whole-body health.

- The gut and the mouth have so many similarities and are in close proximity; they are like "kissing cousins."

- The vast majority of your microbes live in your large intestine.

- Ulcer-causing bacteria can live on dental plaque and can interfere with successful treatments.

- Inflammatory bowel disease is often accompanied by changes to the gut microbiome, the oral microbiome, and immune system responses.

- For stubborn illnesses of the gastrointestinal tract, oral dysbiosis could be a possible hidden cause.

CHAPTER 8

THE ORAL-SYSTEMIC CONNECTION

The mouth is a "mirror of health or disease"
and it may be an early indicator of disease
in other tissues and organs in the body.
—Surgeon General's Report on Oral Health, 2000

Kissing, a pretty smile, great teeth...there are so many reasons to love the mouth. On the other hand, a sick mouth can be a real turn-off. It turns out that there is more to these first impressions than meets the eye. The mouth tells us *a lot* about a person's whole-body health. It can be an indicator of health or disease elsewhere in the body. As we discussed in Chapter 6, dysbiosis in the mouth can cause cavities, gingivitis, periodontal disease, and bad breath. In the US, nearly 50 percent of people over the age of 30 have periodontal disease.[117] But dysbiosis of the oral microbiome doesn't just spell trouble for the mouth—it also can lead to a domino effect of problems at distant sites, including the heart, gut, and joints.

THE LINK BETWEEN ORAL AND HEART HEALTH

Heart disease is the number one killer in the United States. Since gum disease is highly associated with heart disease, it makes sense to address oral health as a way to promote cardiovascular health. Inflammation is a critical underlying disease process in both atherosclerosis and periodontal disease, as inflammation and dysbiosis in the oral cavity can spill over into the blood-stream. This could cause injury and damage to artery walls and contribute to the development of heart disease.

One of the most astounding discoveries is that oral pathogenic bacteria have been found in atherosclerotic plaques in the cardiovascular system. Atherosclerotic plaques are basically clots, or scabs, on the inside lining of blood vessels. If they get displaced, they can block blood vessels and cause a stroke or heart attack.[118] So, the harmful substances involved in heart disease can actually contain oral pathogens like *P. gingivalis*, discussed in Chapter 6. A list of oral bacteria in heart disease plaques can be found on page 158.

> *By balancing the oral microbiome, you are treating systemic disease.*

When people with periodontal disease get treatment, their blood tests for inflammation normalize and indicators of heart disease go away. And that's not all. People who don't keep up with brushing and flossing their teeth are more likely to have high inflammatory markers in their blood and they have a higher risk of heart disease. In fact, brushing and flossing your teeth can immediately reduce your risk of future heart attacks. Get back on the wagon with brushing, flossing, and dental check-ups and *presto!*, you have low risk of heart disease again. It is uncanny.[119, 120]

What Is Atherosclerosis?

Atherosclerosis is a type of heart disease that narrows and hardens the arteries due to plaque build-up on the artery walls. When the arteries are filled with "junk" and stiffen up, they can't pump blood and it can block blood flow to the heart and other parts of the body. Inflammation is a central feature of atherosclerosis and plaque build-up.[121] Harmful inflammatory chemicals can put little nicks or injuries in the lining of the blood vessels. LDL, sometimes called the "bad" cholesterol, starts to stick to the blood vessel walls, which forms plaque. It goes on to attract immune cells and free radicals, which worsen the plaque production. The final result is plaque made of lipids, immune cells, and scar tissue covering the blood vessel walls. This stiffens the blood vessels so they can no longer pump blood smoothly. When a plaque breaks open, clots can form, blocking blood flow to critical areas of the body, or even causing a stroke or heart attack.

BACTEREMIA AND "LEAKY MOUTH"

What are oral microbiota doing in the circulatory system, anyway? They simply jump on the blood superhighway. In Chapters 3 and 4, we talked about the oral mucosa being permeable and fragile. It tries to keep bad stuff out and let good stuff in. But it is porous, not air tight. For this reason, bacteria can spread from the mouth to the heart through the bloodstream.

Bacteria and chemicals can get through the oral mucous membrane and into the blood on a regular and constant basis. A high amount of bacteria measured in the blood is called "bacteremia." Every time you brush your teeth, get a tooth pulled, or even chew your food, your blood is hit with a flood of oral bacteria.[122] Well, it may not be every single time. The original study from 1954 showing this phenomena saw it occur with 40 percent of periodontal treatments, 35 percent of tooth extractions, 24 percent of brushing teeth, and 17 percent of chewing.[123]

Remember from Chapter 5 that most oral bacteria are beneficial and friendly. But if you have oral dysbiosis, you are effectively sending undesirable bugs coursing through your veins. Something else to know about bacteremia is that the body clears it. I think bacteremia is just a normal fact of life. But bacteremia could be much, much worse in people who have bleeding, puffy, sore gums or "leaky mouth," which we talked about in Chapter 4. Knowing that the oral microbiome has such ready access to the whole body makes it plausible that microbial imbalances and inflammation in the oral cavity could have real impacts on the rest of the system.

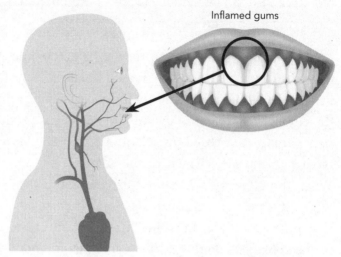

Inflamed gums

Figure 8.1: Blood supply from the heart to the mouth. Note that major arteries go from the heart to the mouth. Blood returning from the mouth has direct access to the heart, which then pumps blood elsewhere in the body.

HOW ORAL PATHOGENS MIGHT CAUSE HEART DISEASE

One popular hypothesis to explain how oral disease leads to heart disease is that periodontal disease causes low-grade inflammation in the bloodstream. Remember that periodontal disease is an out-of-control inflammatory reaction to oral dysbiosis. Red, inflamed gums are like an open, weeping wound that releases high levels of inflammatory biological weapons. If you recall from our discussion in Chapter 4, the immune system is a force to be reckoned with, launching highly toxic chemical and biological warfare against overgrown oral bacteria. The large area of inflamed wound tissue, together with excessive levels of oral bacteria and frequent episodes of bacterial surges in the blood, can lead to low-grade chronic inflammation in the body, damaging the cardiovascular system.[124, 125]

Another hypothesis for how the oral microbiome influences heart health is that pathogenic oral bacteria from the mouth invade the bloodstream and then directly damage the walls of the circulatory system. The oral pathogens can produce toxins that damage the blood vessels and trigger inflammation (or biological warfare), which further damage the blood vessels. When the blood vessels cannot expand and contract to pump blood, it leads to atherosclerosis. Some experts have suggested that pathogenic oral microbes are involved in the instability of these plaques. Perhaps they make plaque more dangerous because a dislodged plaque can cause a clot, heart attack, or stroke. Five periodontal pathogenic bacteria that are involved in heart disease are *Aggregatibacter actinomycetemcomitans*, *Porphyromonas gingivalis*, *Tannerella forsythia*, *Treponema denticola*, and *Fusobacterium nucleatum*.[126]

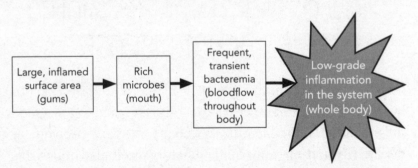

Figure 8.2: This figure illustrates one hypothesis for how oral dysbiosis can spiral out of control and cause disease in the cardiovascular system. In periodontal disease, oral bacteria grow out of control and the immune system launches a powerful, but ineffective, attack. A large area of inflamed gums, high levels of oral bacteria, and frequent surges of bacteria through the bloodstream can produce low-grade, chronic inflammation, which can damage the cardiovascular system and other organ systems.[127]

High-Sensitivity C-Reactive Protein

If inflammation is a central feature of heart disease, then a test that monitors inflammation would be very useful. A biological marker in blood, called high-sensitivity C-reactive protein (hs-CRP), can measure your systemic inflammation. Hs-CRP is released in the blood in response to infection, inflammation, or trauma and is widely used to monitor various inflammatory states. CRP tests are often used to measure a person's risk of heart disease. Blood hs-CRP is often high in heart disease and in periodontal disease and can decrease into the normal range after successful treatments.[128] Hs-CRP can be an important test for determining whole body disease as a result of oral dysbiosis. It's a routine and convenient lab test and can help you monitor inflammation in your body (see more on this in Chapter 9). Hs-CRP is also called CRP, which was the original test name, until it was upgraded to be "high sensitivity." The only difference between hs-CRP and CRP is the sensitivity. Hs-CRP can measure inflammation at much lower levels and therefore has a lower reference range. Use the physician-dentist letter on page 159 if you want to make sure your oral health isn't revving up your inflammation.

HEART HEALTH BENEFITS OF THE ORAL MICROBIOME

The oral microbiome can cause trouble when it is out of balance, but your oral microbiome can also promote heart health. Did you know that your oral bacteria can lower your blood pressure? Bacteria that live in your mouth help you make a chemical called nitric oxide. Nitric oxide plays a critical role in your cardiovascular system to help relax and open the pipes that transport your blood—when your blood vessels are relaxed, blood can flow more smoothly. The result is healthy blood pressure and low risk of heart disease, heart attacks, and strokes. It's good stuff.

Brush your teeth. Your heart will thank you for it.

And our oral bacteria help us make about 25 percent of our total daily needs of nitric oxide by processing foods such as leafy greens and beets.[129] In one experiment, when the participants used antiseptic mouthwash to kill off some of the oral microbiota, the bacteria could no longer help with nitric oxide production, and blood pressure increased! It really makes you think twice about killing your oral microbes with antiseptic mouthwash—that is one reason I don't recommend antiseptic mouthwashes often. The bugs that help lower blood pressure by creating nitric oxide are listed on page 157.

Oral microbiota detected in atherosclerotic plaques include Streptococcus species, Veillonella species, Neisseria species, and the periodontal pathogens *P. gingivalis*, *F. nucleatum*, and *T. forsythia*. Notice that some of these are normal oral bacteria like Streptococcus species. In addition, *S. sanguinis, P. gingivalis, T. denticola*, and *A. actinomycetemcomitans* (the latter three are periodontal pathogens) were found in unstable plaques or clots in patients who had heart attacks.[130]

RHEUMATOID ARTHRITIS

As if oral dysbiosis harming your heart health weren't enough, oral dysbiosis can harm your joints, too. Rheumatoid arthritis (RA) is an autoimmune inflammatory joint disease that eventually destroys a joint and its function. Autoimmune diseases, like rheumatoid arthritis, are examples of what happens when the immune system becomes confused and launches an attack against the host by mistake. It's kind of like a guard dog who gets confused and accidentally bites its owner. In rheumatoid arthritis, the joints are on fire because the immune system is attacking them. Over time, the powerful biological and chemical weapons of the immune system do serious damage to the knee, finger, or hip joints of someone with RA. It damages cartilage and bone and even deforms the joints. Does this sound a little bit like periodontal disease? It's no coincidence. RA and periodontal disease cause similar inflammatory processes and immune system damage to bones and tissues.[131, 132]

The association between RA and periodontal disease is not as strong as the one between cardiovascular disease and periodontal disease, but there are still a lot of compelling similarities. People with RA have a much higher chance of having periodontal disease. If you have rheumatoid arthritis, you are more likely to have bleeding gums, gingivitis, and deep tooth pockets, which are characteristic of periodontal disease. And when rheumatoid patients are treated for periodontal disease, sometimes their joints feel much better afterward and their systemic markers of inflammation calm down (like hs-CRP, on page 105). This isn't a new phenomenon. Even Hippocrates saw arthritis improve after pulling a patient's tooth.[133, 134]

One of the most definitive red flags is that certain pathogenic oral microbes have been found in the fluid surrounding sick joints of people with RA! The fact that oral bacteria can leave their homes in the mouth and reach the joints and set up shop there seems otherworldly. But if anyone can work magic tricks like that, it would be bacteria. Other oral bacteria found in diseased joints were *Prevotella intermedia, P. gingivalis, Fusobacterium nucleatum,* and *Serratia proteamaculans.*[135]

There are a lot of questions about how this happens and what this means. One interesting theory is that a certain oral bacteria that is high in periodontal disease has the ability to make a special kind of protein that activates rheumatoid arthritis. Citrullinated peptides are a kind of altered protein that seem to trigger inflammatory responses in autoimmune diseases, such as RA. In the vast majority of RA patients (70 percent), their immune system is attacking these citrullinated peptides.[136] In fact, citrullinated peptides are such a key factor to the disease that they are used to diagnose it and monitor treatment. It just so happens that *P. gingivalis*, a common oral pathogen, carries an enzyme that can citrullinate, or alter, proteins, which then provoke an immune attack.[137, 138]

Almost 2,500 years ago, Hippocrates, the father of medicine, wrote that pulling a person's tooth could cure arthritis.

Other immune and inflammatory mechanisms, bone destruction processes, and similar genetic underpinnings could also explain the association between RA and periodontal disease. While there is still more to understand about rheumatoid arthritis and oral health, for now it is safe to say that taking care of oral health could help reduce inflammation, keep bad bugs under control, and protect joints from disease. Also, for a person with rheumatoid arthritis, keeping on top of oral health and balancing the oral microbiome could help reduce joint pain and inflammation.

Connecting the Dots

Does your dentist ask about your heart health? Does your primary care doctor ask about your gum health? Or even your gut health, for that matter? These artificial divisions in medicine and dentistry give us the idea that all of our organs work in isolation. On the contrary, they are *all connected*. Your oral health is a factor in your gut health, and your heart health, and more. My dentist says, "It is not a closed system." The mouth is a gateway to the body and it shows.
Use the letter on page 159 to help your physician and dentist collaborate on your oral-systemic health.

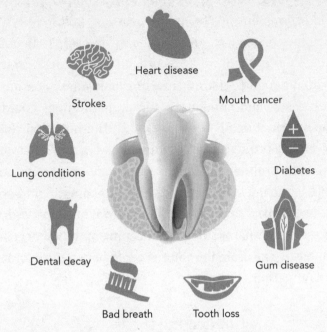

Figure 8.3: Gum disease and oral dysbiosis can manifest as many other conditions in the body.

A Note of Caution

I want to urge caution with pointing the finger at pathogenic oral bacteria as the cause of heart disease or rheumatoid arthritis. Yes, pathogenic bacteria from the oral cavity were detected in heart disease plaques and in diseased joints. It's important to know. However, *just one bug is not the problem.* It is the whole microbial shift in the oral microbiome that allows a pathogen to rise to power. When oral dysbiosis occurs, a whole slew of negative things happen in the microbial communities, at the oral mucosal barrier, and with the immune system. Certain pathogens rising to power and creating havoc (like *P. gingivalis*) cannot simply be solved with a round of antibiotics. It's not a one-bug-one-disease model anymore. If you learn anything in this book, please learn that antibiotics are good for serious, isolated infections but not for bigger, chronic problems with the microbiome. Instead, if you have heart disease or rheumatoid arthritis, then you will want to cultivate a healthier oral microbiome that protects you and pushes bad guys out. You want to fortify a stronger oral barrier that keeps bad guys out of the systemic circulation. You want to shift the microbial ecology from one that promotes disease to one that promotes systemic health. Diet, probiotics, dental hygiene, and other treatments can help to grow a healthy garden of good bacteria that protect you from the likes of periodontal pathogens like *P. gingivalis*. A comprehensive list of oral microbiome solutions can be found in Chapter 9.

Heart Disease Begins in the Mouth

A 62-year-old woman named Linda went to her doctor for her annual check-up. Dr. Ellie Campbell did the usual battery of tests on Linda, including blood sugar, cholesterol, and hs-CRP. Linda said she was feeling fine and didn't report any major issues with her health. Linda's lab tests came back and she had high levels of hs-CRP in her blood, which suggested that she had an infection or another source of inflammation in her body. Once Dr. Campbell found out Linda had high hs-CRP, she tested Linda's oral bacteria with the MyPerioPath test from OralDNALabs (see an example in Chapter 9, Figure 9.1). She wanted to see if Linda's marker of heart disease might have its origin in the mouth.

Linda's oral DNA test showed elevations of eight different periodontal pathogens, including *T. denticola* and *P. intermedia*. Dr. Campbell started Linda on a protocol to improve her oral health by decreasing the unhealthy microbes in her mouth. Dr. Campbell recommended Linda use a stainless steel tongue scraper before brushing her teeth. She told Linda to add GUM soft picks to her flossing regimen. She also suggested that Linda add two drops of frankincense essential oil to her Waterpik.

When Linda came back for her next annual exam the following year, her hs-CRP had dropped by half. However, it was still elevated. Since her hs-CRP still hinted that there was unchecked inflammation, Dr. Campbell told Linda to continue on her protocol with the tongue scraper, the GUM soft picks, and the frankincense essential oil in the Waterpik. But this time she told Linda to start taking ProbioMax DDS (Xymogen) once per day, at bedtime. ProbioMax DDS is a chewable probiotic that contains the beneficial oral bacterium *S. salivarius* DSM 14685.

When Linda did her testing in the following year, everything looked much better. Her hs-CRP was much improved and within the normal range. Likewise, her oral microbial DNA looked much better. Her pathogenic bacteria decreased by half. Where there were eight different bacteria present in her first test, her follow-up test showed only four.

Linda's marker of inflammation was much better after treating her oral health and this corresponded with an improvement in her oral microbiome. Linda's risk of heart disease was reduced by restoring oral microbiome balance.

Dr. Campbell summed it up beautifully: "The moral of this story is that when CRP is high, always check the mouth with an oral bacteria test. Heart disease begins in the mouth! Treat the mouth and you can treat the inflammation. Reduce the inflammation and you reduce the risk for stroke and heart attack."

DIABETES

The state of your gums seems to reflect on the state of your heart and your joints. But did you know it also can influence your sugar metabolism? Much like heart disease, there is a significant bidirectional association between type 2 diabetes and periodontal disease. Bidirectional means that having diabetes makes you more likely to develop gum disease, and having gum disease makes you more likely to develop diabetes. Here's another way to look at it: Get your blood sugar under control and your gum disease goes away; boost your oral health and you can better control your blood sugar.[139]

Again, we don't have a firm explanation for this uncanny relationship. We know that having diabetes means your risk of having gum disease is three times greater than if you didn't have diabetes. And treatments for periodontal disease can improve measures of blood sugar, but not always. Since both diabetes and periodontal disease are characterized by excess inflammation, a common gene that alters immune function, the HLA genotype, may explain why both conditions show up together.[140]

Another theory for the close relationship of these two conditions is that in diabetes, the immune system is damaged from advanced glycation end products (AGEs), which are basically toxic sugar molecules (think of burnt sugar in the bottom of your oven). The damaged sugars cause the immune system to malfunction. Immune cells become hyper aggressive and hostile against bacterial biofilm, launching a violent assault. Remember that periodontal disease is a disease of an overactive immune response against oral dysbiosis. It destroys gums and bone, and can cause teeth to loosen and fall out. AGEs can damage tissues and slow down wound healing, further contributing to periodontal disease.[141]

The microbiome can affect metabolism, weight, and diabetes. Scientists have noticed patterns of gut microbes in people who are obese or lean. Firmicutes phyla are higher than Bacteroidetes phyla in people who are obese. Lean people have the opposite pattern. When researchers changed the participants' diets, their Bacteroidetes increased, Firmicutes decreased, and they lost weight. While most of the research is on the gut microbiome, I wouldn't be surprised if we find out one day that our oral microbes influence our weight and metabolism. We already know they can affect our blood sugar!

SO, NOW WHAT DO I DO?

It is sometimes unbelievable that something as small and seemingly insignificant as the mouth could have such a huge impact on heart health, joint health, blood sugar control, metabolism, and more. Researchers are hard at work trying to discover how and why the oral microbiome is so pivotal to overall health. For now, we need to shift away from the outdated model of trying to kill off a single oral pathogen with antibiotics. Instead, balance and repair your oral microbes to improve gut health, reduce inflammation, promote heart health, boost your metabolism, and reduce painful joints. In the next chapter, I will give you practical action steps and resources to get your oral microbiome, and whole body, in tip-top shape.

Takeaways

- Gum disease increases the chances of having heart disease and diabetes.

- Gum disease is common in people with rheumatoid arthritis.

- Excessive inflammation is a common theme in gum disease, heart disease, rheumatoid arthritis, and diabetes.

- Every time you brush, eat, or get a dental cleaning, a surge of bacteria courses through your bloodstream, a phenomenon called bacteremia.

- Oral bacteria can take a ride in the bloodstream and land in far-off sites.

- Forget the outdated model of one-bug-one-disease; cultivate healthy bacterial communities to ward off disease.

- Hs-CRP is a routine blood test that tells you your levels of inflammation; it is used to measure the risk of heart disease.

- If you have any of the conditions listed in this chapter, work on optimizing your oral micro-biome and oral health.

CHAPTER 9

ORAL MICROBIOME SOLUTIONS

"The doctor of the future will give no medicine but will interest his patients in the care of the human frame, in diet, and in the cause and prevention of disease."

—Thomas Edison

You have the power to keep your oral microbiome healthy. You can also do things to heal your oral microbiome if it is sick. One of the great things about the mouth is that it is easy for you to access. You can promote health from the inside and from the outside. For instance, your diet influences your oral microbiome (and every other cell in your body, for that matter). When you change your diet, you are improving your microbiome from the inside. You can also directly affect the bugs in your mouth with probiotic toothpastes, by avoiding mouthwash, and more.

The major ways you can impact your oral microbiome are through:

- Diet

- Nutrition

- Dental hygiene

- Balancing your microbes with supplements or medications

- Lowering inflammation

- Healing mouth tissue

- Boosting your immune system

In this chapter, I will also tell you about the cutting-edge tests available to find out what bugs are living in your mouth. I will list resources to help you find an integrative and functional medicine doctor to work with in your area. In Chapters 7 and 8, you learned that the mouth is intimately interconnected with the rest of the body, so it could be that your oral microbiome is not the root cause of your health problems. On the contrary, you may have a disease process going on elsewhere in your body that is just producing symptoms in the mouth. Therefore, you may need to work with a clinician to address other problem areas first, in order to restore health to your mouth. Continue reading about the many treatments and resources available to help you optimize your oral microbiome.

*"Every time you eat or drink you are
either feeding disease or fighting it."*
—Heather Morgan, MS

DIET

Your diet is one of the most powerful ways to influence your microbiome. Have you heard the adage "You are what you eat"? It might be more appropriate to say instead, "You are what your bugs eat." All of our bugs have evolved alongside us for millennia. They eat what we eat. Bacteria eat the break-down products of protein, fiber, sugar, fats, and plants, just like we do. Your microbiome likes plant-based foods. One of the most powerful ways to shift your microbiome is to eat more plant-based foods and fiber. Prebiotics, found in these foods, are literally bacteria food. The more prebiotics you eat, the more you feed your good bugs, and the happier you and your bugs are. Take a look back at Chapter 5, page 61, to learn more about prebiotics. Examples of prebiotic foods are chicory root, Jerusalem artichoke, banana, and whole grain breakfast cereal.

If you have trouble eating lots of vegetables and fruits, you can also take prebiotics in a powder form. Nutritional supplements contain these common prebiotics: galacto-oligosaccharides, inulin, and larch arabinogalactan. Klaire Labs has BiotaGen and Designs for Health has PaleoGreens and PaleoReds (available through a practitioner). Another popular prebiotic supplement is SunFiber, which contains guar gum and is tasteless, colorless, and odorless.

For a comprehensive guide about the diet that promotes oral health, see *The Dental Diet*, by Dr. Steven Lin. It includes a step-by-step meal plan with recipes. Books that tell you how to feed your gut microbiome will apply equally well to feeding your oral microbiome, too.

Breastfeeding

In our first days and months of life, we are given milk, even before we eat a whole foods diet. Breastmilk is by far the *best* milk for an infant's microbiome, as we discussed earlier. It is chock-full of mother's good bacteria, the prebiotics that feed those bacteria, and immune boosters, among many other nutritional and health benefits. Breastfeeding provides all of the nutrients needed to build strong teeth and nourish the mouth. It also helps develop the jaw, the nasal cavity, and alignment of the teeth.[142]

Breastmilk gives a child a foundation of healthy bacteria that will colonize the gut, the mouth, the skin, and the rest of the body. Nature has designed a magnificent system whereby a mother passes on her microbiome to her child through vaginal childbirth and breastfeeding (see Chapter 5). Antibiotics, C-section births, and infant formula interfere with the process of transferring mother's microbiome to her child. These things should be avoided, when at all possible.

Despite our best efforts, however, children are born by C-section and/or can't breastfeed at alarmingly high rates. There are some things you can do to simulate the microbiome transfer that normally happens during vaginal birth and breastfeeding.

One technique to restore a baby's microbiome after C-section delivery is called vaginal seeding, whereby gauze is placed into the mother's vagina where it absorbs the mother's vaginal fluid (and good bacteria). When the baby is delivered, the gauze is removed and then brushed over the newborn's mouth, nose, and skin. A very small study showed that vaginal seeding "rescued" the C-section infant's microbiome[143] and restored it so that it more closely resembles that of babies born vaginally. Pretty incredible! I did it with my daughter. Some doctors discourage this practice, saying that there is not enough evidence to support it. They believe pathogenic microbes in the mother's vaginal fluids could present harm to the newborn. Instead, they encourage at least six months of breastfeeding to overcome the depletion of microbes caused by the C-section birth.

Mothers who can't breastfeed should consider using donor human milk. Human breast milk is actually recommended by the American Academy of Pediatricians for all premature infants because it reduces the risks of blindness, blood infections, gut infections, and death in these vulnerable babies. When breast milk isn't available, they recommend pasteurized human donor milk over formula. Dairy and soy infant formula can't even touch the sublime benefits to health and the microbiome of human milk for our babies.

And even before birth, you can optimize your microbiome so that it's in tip-top shape for your baby. Take probiotics during pregnancy to help boost your good bacteria and gut function. A healthy diet low in sugar and refined carbs, and rich in vegetables and fruits will help grow your healthy bacteria. You can offer the same kinds of healthy foods to your baby when he or she starts eating solid foods. Don't give them sugar or cereals, but instead veggies and fruit to help them cultivate a garden of beneficial bacteria. Avoid antibiotics before, during, and after pregnancy, when possible. Chronic ear infections in babies can be a sign of food sensitivities, so exercise caution when introducing allergenic foods into your baby's diet (such as wheat, dairy, corn, and soy). Limiting allergenic foods can help to reduce infections and unwanted antibiotics.

Get Rid of Your Sweet Tooth

A diet high in sugar and refined carbohydrates (which turn to sugar quickly) is like feeding your microbiome junk food. Examples of foods high in sugar and refined carbs are crackers, bread, pasta, cereal, baked goods, cakes, cookies, chips, sweets, and white rice. They're not good for you and they're not good for your microbes, either. Sugar and refined carbohydrates can cause harmful bacteria to flourish and take over. Instead, you should eat complex carbohydrates. Complex carbs are found in beans, sweet potatoes, oatmeal, whole wheat, brown rice, and more. Because they take longer for the body to break down, they don't act like a sugar jolt to your system.

Cutting sugar and packaged foods out of your diet will help to balance Candida or other fungi in your mouth. Fungi and yeasts (a type of fungus) like sugar. If high Candida is a problem in the mouth (or in the gut), you can lower it by cutting foods out of your diet that are high in fungus, such as bread, cheese, beer, corn, and nuts. When you eat these foods, you are increasing fungal levels in your mouth and gut. Some people have trouble keeping their fungal microbiome in balance. They may have vaginal yeast infections, jock itch, athlete's foot, a white coating on their tongue (thrush), or other symptoms of fungal over-growth. These people often benefit from an "anti-Candida diet" that is low in sugar, starch, and the foods listed above, as well as mushrooms and vinegar.

See if you can give up sugar, soda, and processed foods. Sugar does nothing good for your mouth or your body. Instead, use natural sweeteners like stevia leaf and xylitol from the birch tree. You can also try monk fruit. These are sweeteners that will not cause dysbiosis. In fact, xylitol, which tastes a lot like sugar, actually *fights* cavities. Stevia and xylitol have the added bonus that they are healthy sweeteners for people with diabetes or who are trying to lose weight.

If you have extreme sugar cravings, you may have a serious dysbiosis. Bacteria and yeast can take over, causing you to crave sugar. Intense sugar cravings can also be a sign of hormonal imbalance or problems with your metabolism. Consider finding an integrative and functional medicine practitioner to help figure out the root cause of sugar cravings so you can start making healthier food choices.

Instead of eating sugars and refined carbohydrates, choose vegetables, fish, meats, eggs, fruit, and whole grains. Try to cook at home more frequently. Green tea and other herbal teas also are good food for our bacteria because they contain polyphenols, a natural product in plants that bacteria like to eat. Green tea also fights cancer. Whole foods are what our microbiomes have been accustomed to eating for millennia, and they are better for us, too!

Fruits should be eaten sparingly. Use whole fruit to satisfy your sweet tooth instead of fruit juices, foods with added sugar, or packaged foods that are high in refined carbohydrates. While certainly some fruits are acidic, acidic fruits are not the major cause of high acid in the mouth. Instead, make sure to eliminate other causes of high acid in the mouth, like sugar, fruit juice, and soda.

When you eat fermented foods such as sauerkraut, kimchi, and kombucha, you are eating good bacteria that will impact your mouth and gut. Keep in mind that pasteurization kills good bacteria. So look for these products that have not been treated. Making your own fermented foods is another option. However, exercise caution because we don't know all of the microorganisms that grow in these fermented concoctions. Things like sauerkraut and kimchi have been eaten for millennia, so fermenting foods is not dangerous, but it would be better to buy it (or starter cultures) from a trusted source.

Many people think yogurt is a good dietary probiotic. I don't agree. The first problem is any flavored yogurt has a lot of refined sugar in it. That's not good for your bacteria and yeast. Secondly, yogurt doesn't deliver high doses of probiotics, just lower doses. To fully benefit from the perks of probiotics, you will likely need higher doses that are typically found in supplements. Unsweetened yogurt is certainly a healthy food, but I wouldn't rely totally on it to provide your body with all of the beneficial bacteria that you need (take a look at Balancing Your Microbes on page 131).

NUTRITION

Your body requires a long list of vitamins, minerals, amino acids, fatty acids, and carbohydrates in order to stay healthy. Every cell of the body, including those of the mouth, needs these nutrients to function at its best. Your diet should include all of these life-sustaining nutrients. A healthy diet discourages cavities, helps build enamel, prevents tooth break-down, and fortifies the immune system. It nourishes the oral mucosa so that it can defend itself and heal rapidly. Certain nutrients can promote saliva production, which is critical for oral health. Unfortunately, even an organic, whole foods, healthy diet may not deliver all these nutrients to meet your body's demands. Nutritional supplementation may be needed.

Pretty much everyone needs a foundational nutrition plan that includes a diet of healthy proteins, complex carbohydrates, essential fatty acids (including linolenic and alpha-linoleic acids), plenty of vegetables, and supplements, including a multi-vitamin-mineral and a probiotic (see specific recommendations on page 131). If you have oral dysbiosis, then these nutritional recommendations are all the more important for you. In addition, certain nutrients have been shown to specifically benefit the mouth. And keeping the tissue in the mouth and the teeth healthy helps keep your oral microbiome healthy. The following nutrients are recommended for oral health:

- B vitamins
- Calcium
- Copper
- Coenzyme Q10 (CoQ10)
- Folate
- Magnesium
- Phosphorous

- Potassium
- Vitamin A
- Vitamin C
- Vitamin D
- Vitamin E
- Vitamin K2
- Zinc

Vitamins D and A are necessary for healthy enamel on teeth. Calcium and other minerals help build teeth and keep teeth strong, while vitamins D and K help direct tooth formation. Low protein, iron, or zinc can slow down saliva production, worsening nutrition in the mouth and leaving the mouth defenseless against infection. If you don't have good levels of folate (the synthetic version is called "folic acid"), you are more likely to develop periodontal disease. Deficiencies of B vitamins can cause inflammation of the lining of the mouth and tongue, a burning sensation of the tongue, and more.[144]

Antioxidants like CoQ10 and vitamins A, D, E, and C help protect the mouth from the dangers of smoking, tobacco products, and alcohol consumption. Some studies have shown that people with gum disease and bleeding gums have low levels of CoQ10 in their gums. CoQ10 treatment can reduce gingivitis and bleeding gums, as can Vitamin C. You can deliver these nutrients directly to teeth and gums by using a toothpaste such as Revitin Prebiotic Toothpaste, which contains CoQ10, vitamins C, D, K, calcium carbonate, and prebiotics.[145, 146, 147]

If you eat a diet of junk food, fast food, or lots of packaged foods, you may not have good nutrition. If you don't eat the rainbow of vegetables, you may be malnourished. If you have a chronic illness, your body may be drained of vital nutrients. If you weren't breastfed, you might have had a poor nutritional start. If you suspect that you have a weak nutritional foundation, you should see a clinician who can test your levels and replenish these fundamental nutrients with diet and supplements (see Finding an Integrative and Functional Healthcare Practitioner on page 143). Your oral health—and perhaps your bodily health—depends on it.

DENTAL HYGIENE

I am a big fan of the oral microbiome. But our oral bacteria can overgrow and become imbalanced, or dysbiotic. If we never brushed our teeth, we would have tons of bacteria living in our mouths. And as much as I like good bacteria, in high numbers they will probably cause gum disease and cavities. The trick isn't to kill off all bacteria or to let them grow wildly out of control, but to keep them in balance. Since the advent of dental hygiene, we have tools at our disposal to keep our bacteria from growing out of control. For someone with oral infections or dysbiosis, antimicrobial treatments and even antibiotics may still be necessary, but we should exercise caution not to kill oral bacteria needlessly.

Dental hygiene physically removes the microorganisms in the mouth. Dental hygiene keeps plaque lower and helps prevent cavities and oral dysbiosis. Studies show that well-off teenagers who brushed their teeth daily with a fluoride-containing toothpaste, had dietary and oral hygiene counseling, fluoride treatments, and regular dental visits since early childhood had a low rate of oral dysbiosis, specifically in the form of cavities.[148]

Brushing teeth affects the oral microbiome and the gut microbiome. When people brushed after every meal, it significantly decreased Candida levels in the saliva and stool, much more than brushing one time per day.[149] Brushing and flossing lowers inflammatory markers in your blood and reduces your risk of heart attacks in real-time.[150] As you saw in the case story from Chapter 8, Dr. Ellie Campbell changed her patient's oral microbiome by recommending a stainless steel tongue scraper before brushing, GUM soft picks, and frankincense oil in the patient's Waterpik.

However, oral hygiene doesn't affect the major players in the oral microbiome. It affects the relative proportions of each bug in the community. Even two human populations with totally different brushing and flossing habits both had the same "core microbiome," as we discussed in Chapter 5. The same 24 bacterial species were found in all participants, and the same 78 species were found in 90 percent of the participants. That's a lot of overlap for people with different dental hygiene habits.

When people stopped all forms of oral hygiene, the bacteria in their mouths skyrocketed after only four days. By day 10 without oral hygiene, everyone in the study had developed moderate to severe gingivitis. When they resumed their normal dental care, they were able to lower the overall amounts of bacteria on their teeth. But the composition of the microbiome on their teeth did not bounce back to baseline, even after two weeks of renewed oral hygiene. The changes to the tooth microbiome stuck, despite getting back on the dental hygiene wagon.[151] What we do can dramatically affect our microbial populations; even 10 days without brushing can change your microbiome semi-permanently.

Brushing and flossing not only keep the bacteria levels down, they also act as a physical therapy to keep the oral mucosa and gums healthy. My dental hygienist highly recommends a Waterpik water flosser, or water irrigation of gums and teeth. She has seen excellent results, often better than flossing, to keep gums plump, healthy, and strong. These therapies stimulate and strengthen your gum tissue and help the gums stay tight around the teeth, like a suction cup. Healthy, strong gums reinforce the oral mucosa and form a strong defensive barrier, which keeps bad bugs out of the bloodstream where they don't belong. If you want to revisit this, we discussed the barrier and the problems caused by leaky mouth in Chapter 4. The key to oral hygiene is finding the tools that work best for you, both in terms of your daily habits and what therapies make your teeth and gums happy.

Fluoride

In one of my biology classes in college, we were told matter-of-factly that adding fluoride to our water system was one of the greatest public health victories of all time and had dramatically reduced the incidence of cavities. Indeed, dentists use fluoride treatments to strengthen and rebuild teeth. Calcium, found in the tooth's hard hydroxyapatite material, can be swapped out for fluorine, which makes teeth more durable and less susceptible to cavities.

It was only when I started working at an integrative and functional medicine laboratory that I learned that not everyone agreed with my biology professor. Groups of dentists and physicians oppose water fluoridation because of its health risks. In population studies and animal studies, fluoride exposure seems to harm brain development. At the time of writing this, a study came out suggesting that fluoride could be neurotoxic to unborn babies. The more fluoride that pregnant women were exposed to, the more likely their future children were to have ADHD, even years later.[152] Between fluoride in water, toothpaste, food, pharmaceuticals, and other sources, we may be getting much more fluoride than we need. In fact, too much fluoride causes fluorosis, a harmless discoloration or surface pitting on teeth, which has been reported in 41 percent of US teenagers.[153] To fluoridate or not is a hotly debated topic so you will want to do further reading to come to your own conclusion about fluoride, oral health, and overall health. At the minimum, be careful about fluoride exposure during pregnancy and in children.

Smoking

Smoking increases your risk of gum disease, diabetes, heart disease, cancer, obesity, and more. Stop smoking to improve your oral microbiome, decrease oral dysbiosis, and fight disease elsewhere in the body. This is one of the all-time best things you can do for your overall health. Quitting can be extremely difficult. Check with government smoking cessation programs and even your health insurance company for resources and moral support to help you quit.

Healthy Salivary Flow

Perhaps you take saliva for granted, or you just see it as a nuisance. A generous flow of healthy saliva is absolutely essential for a healthy mouth! It is packed with nutrients that feed your teeth and gums. It washes away bacteria so that they don't overgrow. It carries molecules that protect your teeth and gums, raise your immune defenses, and fight infections. Eating a healthy diet and making sure you have good levels of vitamins and minerals will ensure that your saliva can do its job. Drink plenty of water—half of your body weight in ounces each day. Chewing up whole foods can help salivary flow; chewing certain foods such as peanuts, gum, and hard cheeses seems to stimulate saliva production. If you have an autoimmune disease or other illness that causes dry mouth, please see page 143 to find a practitioner that can help you address that condition as well as support your oral health.

If you are a "mouth-breather," it means that you breathe in most of your air through your mouth, instead of your nose. Breathing through your nose is actually a healthier way to breathe. Mouth-breathing can dry up saliva and increase bad breath, cavities, and gum disease. What does that mean? Mouth-breathing contributes to dysbiosis of your oral microbiome. If you notice that you breathe through your mouth by day and have dry mouth when you wake up in the morning, check out resources by Dr. Mark Burhenne, on how to turn around mouth-breathing at askthedentist.com.

BALANCING YOUR MICROBES

Boost Your Good Bugs

The most obvious way to alter your oral microbiome is to encourage good bugs to grow or get rid of bad bugs. You can boost your good bacteria levels by taking probiotics and prebiotics. You feed your good bacteria when you eat a diet rich in plant-based foods and fiber. We will talk about how to remove bad bacteria in the next section.

Probiotics are beneficial bacteria that cause no harm. They can be taken as a pill, powder, or paste. Probiotics can crowd out bad bacteria and help fight infections. They can change the environment of the mouth so that other friendly bacteria can have an easier time growing. They help you shift your microbiome to a healthier balance of bacteria. Fermented foods, such as sauerkraut, kimchi, and kombucha, also contain beneficial bacteria (see Diet on page 119).

There are many great probiotics out on the market now. Most of them are for improving gastrointestinal function. Probiotics taken in a capsule can alleviate symptoms like diarrhea, constipation, bloating, stomach ache, gas, and more. I like Custom Probiotics (available online) and Masters Supplements (available through a practitioner). Take 50 to 300 billion colony forming units per day (CFU/day) to provide your body with a good dose of healthy microbiota. A dose of 50 billion CFU/day is appropriate for maintaining health. A dose of 300 billion CFU/day is appropriate for someone with serious illness related to bacterial imbalance, such as ulcerative colitis. At high doses like 300 billion CFU/day, you should be under the care of a healthcare professional knowledgeable about probiotic therapies.

Some common probiotics, backed up by scientific evidence, to help promote gut health are:[154]

- BioGaia by Everidis Health Sciences

- Culturelle by Valio, Helsinki, Finland/Amerifit Brands, Inc.

- DanActive by Dannon

- VSL #3 by Sigma-Tau Pharmaceuticals, Inc.

Probiotics usually contain Lactobacillus and Bifidobacteria species. Look for brands with a variety of species. These have many great health benefits for the intestines and rest of the body!

We know probiotics do great things for the gut, but what about the mouth? It should be no surprise to you after reading this book: They do great things for the mouth, too! Probiotic supplements for the gums and teeth decrease the numbers of bacteria that cause cavities and they help to get rid of periodontal pathogens (bugs that are thought to cause gum disease). When people with periodontal disease took oral probiotics, they had less bleeding and their gums were healthier and more supple.[155] Probiotics calm down inflammation (the immune system's biological warfare against dysbiosis). They make chemicals that kill off unwanted bacteria. Oral probiotics can stick to teeth and make a place for themselves at the "dinner table," effectively kicking bad bugs out of the picture. They help to kick Candida species out of the mouth, too. If you want to refresh your memory about oral dysbiosis that causes cavities or gum disease, take a look at Chapter 6.

So far, the main probiotics that improve oral health are Lactobacillus species, Bifidobacteria species, and Streptococcus species. Lactobacillus have been estimated to make up approximately 1 percent of the oral commensal flora. The Lactobacillus strains found in saliva are *L. fermentum, L. rhamnosus, L. salivarius, L. casei, L. acidophilus,* and *L. plantarum.*[156]

Oral Probiotic Effect on Cavities, Gum Disease, and Organisms Involved in Cavities (*Streptococcus Mutans*) or Periodontal Disease[157, 158]

ORAL PROBIOTIC SPECIES	HEALTH BENEFITS IN THE MOUTH
Bifidobacteria species	Decreases *S. mutans*
Bifidobacteria lactis	Decreases *S. mutans*
Lactobacillus species	Reduces periodontal pathogens: *P. gingivalis*, *Prevotella intermedia*, and *A. actinomycetemcomitans*
Lactobacillus brevis	Improves gingivitis; improves periodontal disease
Lactobacillus paracasei	Prevents cavities; reduces *S. mutans*; reduces *P. gingivalis*
Lactobacillus plantarum	Reduces *S. mutans*
Lactobacillus rhamnosus GG	Reduces *S. mutans*; reduces oral pathogens; prevents cavities; improves periodontal disease
Lactobacillus reuteri	Reduces *S. mutans*; reduces *Candida*; reduces dental plaque in gingivitis
Lactobacillus salivarius	Reduces *S. mutans*; maintains oral health
Streptococcus salivarius K12	Prevents gum disease; may prevent bad breath
Streptococcus salivarius M18	Prevents gum disease; may prevent bad breath
Weissella cibaria (previously a Lactobacillus species)	Reduces bad breath

Saccharomyces boulardii is a friendly yeast. It is also a probiotic. Since it is a fungus, it's ideally suited to crowd out other, less friendly fungi. Since dysbiosis in the mouth may be fungal as well as bacterial, a combination of probiotics and *S. boulardii* may be needed. A common brand of *S. boulardii* is Florastor by Biocodex, Inc.

If you have dysbiosis in the mouth, consider using a probiotic toothpaste or chewable probiotics. This delivers probiotics directly to your gums, tongue, and teeth. Designs for Health carries PerioBiotic Toothpaste. A study on PerioBiotic Toothpaste showed that it reduced levels of plaque. It also lowered the cavity-causing bacteria, *S. mutans*, after brushing. However, when participants had a high-sugar drink, it blunted the effects of the toothpaste, once again showing that the oral microbiome is an interaction of diet, microbes, and other factors.[159] Other oral probiotics include Prodegin TM from Klaire Labs, which is a chewable probiotic for oral health (they also carry a children's chewable probiotic); TheraBreath carries oral probiotics and probiotic lozenges. GUM PerioBalance is a lozenge designed to prevent gum disease; it contains probiotic strains of *Lactobacillus reuteri*.

Protect your microbiome from antibiotics and dental procedures. Remember to take probiotics during and after any treatment with antibiotics. Also, make sure to take probiotics and the friendly yeast, *S. boulardii*, before and after dental procedures. If you are taking antibiotics, you can still take your probiotics, just take them a few hours apart from each other. This helps your good bacteria recover more quickly after getting wiped out by antibiotics.

Get Rid of Bad Bugs

Sometimes bad bugs grow up and take over, causing an infection. Or a group of bad bugs might be "at the top of the heap"

in a bacterial community, creating imbalance. We call this dysbiosis. There are many treatments—both pharmaceutical and
herbal—that lower bad bugs with the hope of re-establishing a
better microbial balance.

Antibiotics can kill off bad bacteria. They are appropriate to use
in serious or dangerous infections or in infections that don't
respond to more gentle treatments. Above all, use antibiotics
with extreme caution. There is a time and a place for antibiotics,
but our society is coming off of a few-decade bender of over-
dosing antibiotics (see Chapter 2). If your doctor recommends
antibiotics, ask this question: What infection do I have? Be wary
of a doctor who wants to treat a virus or an ear infection with
antibiotics if there is no evidence of a true bacterial infection.

Antibiotics wipe out all bacteria, not just the bad guys. And
research tells us that they *never* go back to normal. Bacteria
do grow back rapidly, however; it's just not back to their prior
pattern. The longer you can go without antibiotics, the better.
But when they are necessary, it helps a lot if you have already
been taking probiotics. You should also take probiotics while
taking antibiotics, and after for a few months, to help restore
your microbiome.

Antimicrobial herbs (or herbal antibiotics) are not as powerful
as pharmaceutical antibiotics. Since each herb has thousands of
plant chemicals, they are more similar to natural whole foods.
They have the added bonus of being effective against some bacteria that are antibiotic resistant. There is some research that
suggests they may not obliterate the good bacteria in the same
way that pharmaceutical antibiotics can. For example, garlic
is an antimicrobial herb that can kill pathogenic bacteria but
promote the growth of beneficial bacteria. Some antimicrobial
herbs are berberine, uva ursi, caprylic acid, garlic, oregano

oil, and olive leaf; the latter four also work against bacteria as well as fungi. You can eat more of these herbs in your diet (like oregano, thyme, garlic) if you are trying to lower dysbiosis, but for an infection or widespread dysbiosis, higher doses are typically needed than what you can get from your food. Brands of antimicrobial herbal formulas, or mixtures of different medicinal herbs, include GI Microb-X, ParaBiotic Plus, Berbemycin, Candicidal, Candicid Forte, GI-Synergy, Candibactin-AR, and Candibactin-BR. You may have heard of treatments to break or bust biofilms as a way to root out and destroy unfriendly gut bacteria. While the idea makes sense, these products are in their infancy and should be used only with a skilled integrative and functional medicine practitioner.

You can treat dysbiosis or infection in the mouth directly using antimicrobial mouthwashes, rinses, or even toothpaste. Again, use caution with mouthwash. It can kill the bacteria in your mouth! If you have a microbial imbalance in your mouth, and haven't been able to correct it with other measures, you can try an antimicrobial toothpaste like Dentalcidin by Bio-Botanical Research or an antimicrobial mouth swish such as Dentalcidin LS, also by Bio-Botanical Research, which also contains nutrients for oral care. Both of these products are based on the company's flagship product, Biocidin, which is an herbal antibiotic for gut dysbiosis. Some clinicians simply prescribe a tea tree oral rinse (from tea tree oil) to cut down bacterial and fungal overgrowth in the mouth (as in Grayson's story in Chapter 6).

Use caution with conventional mouthwash that contains antimicrobial agents like chlorhexidine or cetylpyridinium chloride. Conventional antiseptic mouthwashes contain chlorhexidine, an antimicrobial which lowers the bacteria, spores, and fungi in your mouth. Mouthwashes can also contain essential oils, fluoride, alcohol, or peroxide. They are intended to help control or reduce bacteria involved in bad breath, gingivitis, plaque, and cavities. Perhaps that sounds like a good idea, but we now know that blindly killing our oral microbiome could harm our oral and overall health. Bacteria in our mouths help protect us from infection and lower our blood pressure. If you use mouthwash to help with gum disease, cavities, or bad breath, consider instead changing your diet, using oral probiotics, and even using herbal antimicrobials instead. When patients used chlorhexidine-containing mouthwash, their blood pressure increased.[160] Use antiseptic mouthwash when your dentist orders it, before or after surgery or to manage oral infections, especially when you can't brush daily. Listerine Original is a good option because it does not contain chlorhexidine, but instead essential oils from eucalyptus, mint, and thyme.

LOWERING INFLAMMATION

Gingivitis and other diseases often involve inflammation. Inflammation is like having a chemical and biological weapon spill in the body. It can be a response to an infection or to harmful foods or to high sugar in the blood. Our immune systems and healing mechanisms create inflammation when there is something that needs to be killed, like an infection, or healed, like a wound. Inflammation in small doses is a good thing but too much of it can cause serious illness, pain, and suffering.

Microbial dysbiosis can cause inflammation in the mouth. Balance and repair oral dysbiosis by cutting out sugar, soft drinks, and packaged foods, eating more veggies, taking probiotics, rebuilding your nutrition with vitamins, and work on your dental hygiene. If this doesn't shift your oral inflammation, then you may have a baseline of inflammation in the mouth, unrelated to your microbes.

If you have chronic inflammation in your mouth, you will not be able to foster a healthy oral microbiome. You will have trouble healing and will likely have sores, burning, heat, redness, and/or bleeding in the mouth. There is usually a root cause of inflammation that needs to be uncovered and treated. This can clear the way for a healthier immune system that doesn't overreact. However, until you can get help to find out and treat the root cause of inflammation (see page 45), there are things you can do to try to calm down the chemical and biological warfare.

Aloe vera juice is a cooling, soothing plant product that can calm down inflammation in the mouth. Curcumin, from turmeric, is anti-inflammatory, as is resveratrol, which comes from grapes. Eating a diet low in sugar and high in plant-based foods fights inflammation. Limiting meat intake and choosing grass-fed or free-range meat products can calm inflammation. Omega-3 fatty acids, or fish oil, is a natural anti-inflammatory. One gram per day is appropriate for a healthy person, while 3 grams (or more) per day is appropriate for someone fighting inflammation. Make sure to use a high-quality fish oil, one that has been tested for harmful levels of mercury. The Healthy Dentist brand has a Healthy Gums Antigingivitis Rinse that contains 20 percent aloe vera juice. It also contains herbs that fight bacterial overgrowth and those that promote healing.

HEALING MOUTH TISSUE

Even after you've located the root cause of dysbiosis, changed your diet, started supplements, and started working with a healthcare provider, sometimes your body may need a little help to recover from months or years of illness. My recommendations to heal the oral mucosa come from what we know about healing the gut mucosa. When your oral mucosa is healthy and free of disease and inflammation, your beneficial microbes will also flourish.

A number of nutrients and plant components can help heal tissue. These are often dried and ground up into powders and sold as nutritional supplements. L-glutamine is an amino acid that is consumed heavily by the cells lining the GI tract. It helps with tissue healing by giving the cells fuel. Consider swishing powdered glutamine dissolved in water or aloe juice. Zinc carnosine helps to heal mucosal tissue. And slippery, slimy herbs can coat and protect the lining of the mouth so it can heal. Examples are deglycyrrhizinated licorice (DGL), okra, or slippery elm. Healthy Gums Antigingivitis Rinse from The Healthy Dentist, which includes aloe vera juice, can also help to heal the lining of your mouth.

These powders that are made to help soothe and heal the gastrointestinal tract can be dissolved in water, used as a mouth swish, and then swallowed for mouth and gut benefits. These healing ingredients could be added to a tooth bleaching tray or a mouth guard if you want to soak your gums for a short time. Examples of healing powders include GI Revive by Designs for Health and GlutAloeMine by Xymogen. You will need a medical professional to buy these products. If you can't find one, compare the ingredients in these products to over-the-counter products at your local health food store to find a close match.

Another way to enhance the healing of your mouth lining is by giving up all wheat-containing products for a few months. The main allergenic protein in wheat is gliadin. Gliadin damages the connections between cells in the gut mucosa, breaching the intestinal barrier. Given the way gliadin can harm the gut mucosa, it may do the same thing in the mouth, contributing to leaky mouth (discussed in Chapter 4).[161] Staying away from wheat products may help jumpstart the healing of your oral mucosa.

Mercury

Sometimes toxins in the mouth can spell trouble for oral health. Mercury amalgams, or dental fillings that contain mercury, are commonly used in dentistry and have been for centuries. While a very controversial topic, biological dentists and clinicians practicing integrative and functional medicine are very concerned about mercury causing illness in the mouth and elsewhere in the body. In the mouth, mercury can cause soreness, inflammation, and/or gingivitis. Mercury toxicity symptoms elsewhere primarily affect the brain, including the infamous "mad hatter syndrome," insomnia, fatigue, and poor short-term memory, as well as tremors, gut and kidney disturbances, and a suppressed immune system.[162] If you think mercury or another metal implant is affecting your oral health, find a healthcare practitioner (page 143) to consult further. Urine, blood, and hair mercury tests are available to identify daily exposures to this metal.

BOOSTING YOUR IMMUNE SYSTEM

Your mouth's immune system helps protect you from infection, identify and quarantine bad bugs, give entry to good bugs, and sift harmful molecules from harmless ones. When your immune system is overactive, it can cause inflammation. But when it is weak and worn down, it leaves your mouth defenseless.

Suddenly your mouth is wide open to attack from harmful bugs and toxins from the outside world.

Use probiotics such as Bifidobacteria, Lactobacillus, and *S. boulardii* to fortify the immune system in your mouth (and along your GI tract). You can also take colostrum, which is a precursor to breastmilk that contains immunoglobulins, to raise your immune defenses. As discussed earlier in this book, immunoglobulins, such as sIgA, are defense molecules that can bind and remove toxins and bad bugs while promoting a healthy microbiome. Note that colostrum is usually derived from cow's milk and may not be appropriate for dairy-sensitive individuals. Serum-derived immunoglobulins, like Ortho Molecular's SBI Protect (in pill or powder), provide immune support without traces of dairy or egg.

A healthy diet and lifestyle also contribute to a healthy immune system. A good nutritional program including minerals, vitamins, fatty acids, and protein are important for good immune defenses. Other nutrients and herbs that help you fight infection are zinc, echinacea, vitamin A, vitamin C, and vitamin D. Finally, when you lower your stress levels, you give your immune system a chance to recharge. If you are chronically stressed out, it could be draining your immune defenses and leaving you open to imbalances in the mouth.

In our busy, hustle-bustle culture, it is very challenging to reduce stress. First, eating regularly and sleeping for eight hours a night reduces stress. Cut back at work and get exercise at least four times a week. Some people are so stressed they have to block out down time on their calendars. Take naps. Delegate things to others. You can also work with a practitioner to treat adrenal dysfunction, which can help you rein in your fight-or-flight response. They often give nutritional supplements to nourish the adrenal glands and balance stress hormones.

OTHER THINGS TO CONSIDER WHEN OPTIMIZING YOUR ORAL MICROBIOME

We have talked about the main ways you can optimize your oral microbiome: diet and nutrition, dental hygiene, balancing your bugs, lowering inflammation, healing your mouth, and boosting your immune system. But if there is some other, bigger problem going on in your body, many of these efforts may be in vain! Here are some examples of imbalances that could be causing illness in your mouth.

- Food sensitivities or allergies. Food sensitivities can drain your immune system so that it can't work properly in the mouth.

- Infection. If you have dysbiosis or an infection somewhere else in your body, it could be causing inflammation that stresses your mouth. One of the most likely places for a hidden infection is the gut.

- Hormone imbalances. If your hormones are imbalanced, it could be contributing to a sick mouth. Pregnancy, menopause, or just growing older can disrupt your hormone balance. Stress can throw your hormones out of whack, disturb your wake and sleep cycle, and suppress your immune system. Women may show hormonal imbalance as fatigue, irritability, low libido, hot flashes, insomnia, acne, or weight gain. If oral dysbiosis symptoms crop up with pregnancy, premenstrual syndrome, or menopause, it's more likely to be a hormone imbalance. Men's hormonal imbalance appears as fatigue, low muscle mass, weight gain, and low sex drive.

- Leaky gut. Discussed in Chapter 4, if you have intestinal permeability, your bloodstream is wide open to the harmful molecules of the outside world. Leaky gut means that you don't have good protection from infections and toxins. Your immune system is often confused and overactive, creating a state of inflammation. If you have leaky gut, you may be more likely to have leaky mouth or damage to the oral mucosa.

FINDING AN INTEGRATIVE AND FUNCTIONAL HEALTHCARE PRACTITIONER

Any of the underlying root causes discussed earlier could be a hold-up when trying to get your oral health back on track. The best option is to find a healthcare practitioner in your area who can help you determine what is holding you back from achieving optimum wellness. I highly recommend finding an integrative and functional medicine practitioner to help you address overall health. The Institute for Functional Medicine has an online directory of clinicians. The Kresser Institute has a directory of clinicians that have completed advanced training in functional medicine and ancestral diet and lifestyle. You can also contact some of these specialty clinical laboratories, which will locate doctors in your area: Diagnostic Solutions Laboratory, Genova Diagnostics, Doctor's Data, Great Plains, Meridian Valley Labs, and Dunwoody Labs. If you don't have an integrative and functional medicine doctor in your area, consider consulting with one that does telemedicine, so you don't have to leave home.

Integrative dentists and biological dentists are harder to find but could be a critical partner in getting your oral health on track. Biological dentists treat the whole person. They don't use mercury or fluoride. They are very careful about metal implants, believing that metals in the mouth must be specifically tailored to, or biocompatible with, the patient. They believe the mouth is connected to the whole body. If you have chronic oral dysbiosis, go to the International Academy of Biological Dentistry and Medicine online to find a biological dentist in your area. The International Academy of Oral Medicine and Toxicology can also help point you to a biological dentist near you.

TESTING

Testing is a powerful tool for you and your healthcare practitioners to get to the underlying causes of illness or simply to optimize wellness. Laboratory tests can detect inflammation, dysbiosis, food sensitivities, infections, hormonal imbalances, or leaky gut using a blood, urine, saliva, or stool sample.

If you have problems with oral dysbiosis, gut dysbiosis, or inflammatory conditions like the ones listed in Chapter 8, the top areas to test are:

1. Microbes. There are tests that measure your oral, fecal, and small intestinal microbes. You can also work with your healthcare provider to order urinary organic acids, which can detect bacterial and fungal metabolism.

2. Immune system. Food sensitivity, celiac disease, and leaky gut testing can help you pinpoint why the immune system is malfunctioning.

3. Inflammation. Use hs-CRP to check your overall state of inflammation.

Microbes

You can run a test to measure your oral microbiome. OralDNA Labs measures bugs in the mouth using a saliva specimen. They are using a type of DNA technology called polymerase chain reaction, or PCR, which is far and above better than microbial culture methods. Your dentist or periodontist may also be able to do a culture test on a specimen from your mouth to see what bugs are in the mix.

Keep in mind that this is a new area of dentistry. Some of the testing profiles may be concerned only with "periodontal pathogens" and may not tell you much about your normal oral microbiota. As we discussed earlier, your oral microbiome is unique. There is no established "normal" microbial composition. That means that even when you have dysbiosis of the mouth, it is still more similar to your normal healthy pattern than it is to anyone else's microbiome. And after you get a dental cleaning or a periodontal treatment, your oral microbiome is still closer to your pattern than anyone else's. That means you have to use yourself as a healthy standard for your oral microbiome pattern. Run tests before and after treatment to monitor your improvements.

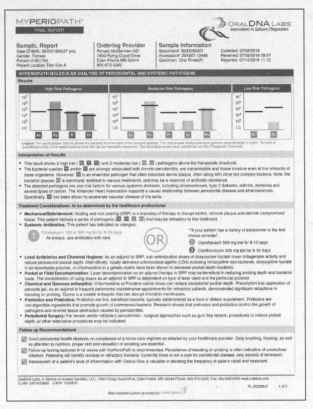

Figure 9.1: Commercial lab testing of oral microbiota using DNA analysis.

Since the mouth and the gut are connected, you may want to consider a stool test to look at your gut microbiome, inflammation, and immune function. Comprehensive stool tests are widely available from these commercial laboratories, through a qualified practitioner: Diagnostic Solutions Lab, Genova Diagnostics, and Doctor's Data. uBiome and Viome also measure gut microbiota with cutting-edge DNA or RNA sequencing. If your doctor runs a test that involves bacterial culture or identifying microbes through a microscope (sometimes called an "Ova and Parasitology" stool test), then you still need a more sophisticated, accurate, and sensitive test that looks at microbial DNA or RNA. If you don't have a clinician to work with, check out My Med Labs, where consumers can order a wide variety of tests on themselves.

Immune System

Tests for food allergies, food sensitivities, and leaky gut are available through many of the laboratories listed in this section. Food sensitivity tests can help you pinpoint which foods may be irritating or draining your immune system. Certain foods, like gluten, can put a person's immune system on red alert. Leaky gut tests help to figure out if your gut mucosa is strong and able to keep large molecules out of the bloodstream. Leaky gut might be an underlying problem in autoimmune diseases and chronic inflammatory conditions.

Inflammation

You can find out your systemic inflammation with a simple, common blood test called hs-CRP (page 105). Ask your healthcare provider to run it along with your cholesterol and blood sugar levels. You can order it without a doctor's prescription in some states.

High CRP says that you have inflammation or infection in the system. It can be a sign of heart disease, oral dysbiosis, or many other conditions. CRP is released in the blood in response to infection, inflammation, or trauma, and is widely used to monitor various inflammatory states. In the Appendix on page 159, you will find a letter by Dr. Mark Burhenne that will help your doctor and your dentist collaborate on your oral health and hs-CRP levels.

After checking that your microbial inhabitants, immune system, and inflammation are all in good shape, you and your healthcare provider may want to test your sex hormones, stress hormones, nutritional status, or even toxicity markers. These tests can help determine if there is another imbalance in your system making it hard for you to get your oral health back on track. Hormonal imbalance can make your mouth sick and unhappy. Poor nutrition can make your gums and teeth weak and prone to infection. Toxicity, from leaky mercury fillings for example, can create inflammation and damage in the mouth.

ORAL MICROBIOME SOLUTIONS FOR ORAL, GUT, AND WHOLE-BODY HEALTH

There are many solutions to oral disease. Some of them are downright simple, like monitoring diet and nutrient intake (although they may be hard to implement). Certain solutions require going to see the dentist or periodontist. Some call for simply taking dietary supplements and natural mouthwashes to help balance the bugs in your mouth, lower inflammation, and heal the lining of your mouth. Other solutions may require partnering with a clinician and running some tests to figure out if something deeper is amiss. But all of these things are possible with the right help, so don't give up!

Takeaways

- You can optimize your oral microbiome from the inside and the outside.

- Your diet is one of the most powerful ways to influence your microbiome.

- Dental hygiene keeps plaque lower and helps prevent cavities and oral dysbiosis.

- Probiotic toothpaste or chewable probiotics deliver probiotics directly to your gums, tongue, and teeth.

- Use antibiotics with extreme caution.

- Hs-CRP tells you how inflamed your body is and can be a clue to a hidden infection.

- The mouth is intimately interconnected with the rest of the body, so a health problem elsewhere could be a hold-up when trying to get your oral health back.

CHAPTER 10

BLIND LUCK

"You know, Hobbes, some days even my lucky rocket ship underpants don't help."
—Bill Watterson, creator of *Calvin and Hobbes*

There are a lot of factors that determine oral health and oral microbial balance. In this book, we've talked about dietary factors such as sugar, refined carbohydrates or packaged foods, plant-based foods, and fiber. Excellent nutrition helps you cultivate a healthy, happy microbiome. I've mentioned that saliva flow, small doses of inflammation, and a healthy working immune system keep your mouth healthy. Whether you were born vaginally or by C-section, and if you were breastfed or bottle-fed, will influence your oral microbiome.

Treatments to reign in bacterial overgrowth in your mouth include brushing, flossing, and regular dental cleanings. You can also rebalance your oral microbiome with probiotics, fermented foods, or even antimicrobial herbs to help take the bacteria down a notch before rebuilding.

But what if none of this works?

Old-fashioned blind luck figures into a healthy mouth, too. Chock it up to bad genetics or a bad assortment of bacteria at birth, but some people do all of the right things and *still* get oral dysbiosis.

An interview with Dr. Mary Ellen Chalmers taught me that doing everything "right" to prevent cavities doesn't work for everyone. There are people who do everything they should do, like eating a healthy diet, brushing, flossing, and seeing the dentist regularly, but they still get cavities. There are people who eat a lot of sugar and simple carbs, don't brush regularly, and don't floss, and they *don't* get cavities! The research backs this up. In populations that have a low rate of cavities and do excellent oral hygiene care, still 1 in 5 people gets cavities.[163] Oral disease doesn't just depend on your oral hygiene. It also depends on your genetics, your diet, and other environmental factors.

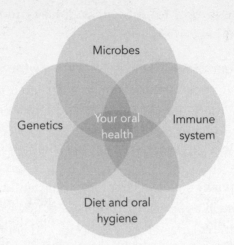

Figure 10.1: Your oral health is the product of interacting forces such as your microbes, your immune system, your environment (such as your diet and oral hygiene), and your genetics.

THE INTERFACE OF MICROBES, IMMUNE FUNCTION, AND ENVIRONMENT

The oral microbiome is the outcome of a conglomeration of different, interconnected factors. Each of these areas influences, and is influenced by, the others. Your genetics came from your parents and can't really be changed. They are the blueprints for every cell in your body and for the system as a whole, but without environmental inputs and a microbiome, genes don't tell us much at all.

As we've discussed through this book, you have at least as many bacterial cells in your body as human cells, if not more. They have their own genes. They make proteins and chemicals and waste products that can affect your immune system, your genes, and even your habits or cravings.

Your immune system works closely together with your microbial inhabitants. If your immune system is irritated or overactive, you will have more inflammation and you may lose tissue and bone because of rampant immune attacks. If your immune system is weak, you are more prone to infections.

Your environment includes your diet, your dental hygiene, and your habits, such as smoking. It influences how your genes are translated into real life and how happy or sad your microbiome is. Your environment, such as the choices you make about your diet or smoking, can boost or weaken your immune system.

Genetics, a good microbiome, and a healthy diet will probably help most people avoid oral dysbiosis. Other people will be susceptible to diabetes and periodontal disease because of their genetics, and perhaps a diet of hamburgers, sandwiches, chips, and soda.

There are plenty of areas to work on to heal and repair your oral microbiota. But there is no guarantee that it will work for everyone, 100 percent of the time. Sometimes, it's just blind luck that gives you a healthy oral microbiome.

Different Oral Microbiomes in One Family

My mom went to a periodontist from the time I can remember. She always said she had "bad teeth." One dentist attributed it to her mother, who smoked while she was pregnant with my mom. Another dentist blamed her "chalky" enamel on powerful antibiotics she was given as a baby when she had pneumonia.

Mom stayed on top of her dental cleanings and dental health, and often had to get root canals and scaling treatments. She flossed every night.

My dad has virtually no issues with his teeth. He goes to the dentist for regular cleanings and also flosses and brushes routinely. He even has all of his wisdom teeth. Like his father, he never needed to remove them because they never gave him trouble. My parents were "health nuts," so we ate a whole-foods diet growing up that was low in sugar.

My brother and I have relatively good oral health. We had childhood cavities, but not many. However, my sister has struggled with oral health over the years. Like my mom, she is more prone to cavities. She has had trouble with her teeth wearing down.

We were all breastfed, vaginally born babies. We ate similar diets through childhood. I would venture to say we all have a similar oral microbiome since we would have inherited it from our mother and father, and we were living in the same home, eating a similar diet. But at the end of the day, our oral health was not identical. Was there a different genetic predisposition? Were there different microbes at play? Was nutrition or immune function to blame? There is much we don't yet know about the oral microbiome, and until there is a more scientific explanation, I'll say that some people have good oral health simply because they are lucky.

There is so much we don't know and we don't understand. The study of the oral microbiome is in its infancy. Remember, only 57 percent of the oral microbiome is even named and characterized. I write this chapter to acknowledge and validate the people who struggle with oral disease and dysbiosis even when they have stellar dental hygiene, eat a sugar-free and whole-foods diet, and tend to their nutrition and their microbiomes.

To those people, I would say: While we can't change our genetics or our pasts, we *can* change our environment and our microbes. Keep working to promote a healthy microbiome by following the recommendations in Chapter 9. Keep looking for the unique combination of things that work best to optimize *your* oral health. Find a skillful doctor and dentist who can work with you to find the root causes of your symptoms. Use laboratory testing to establish your baseline and monitor your progress. And look beyond the mouth for disease processes elsewhere in the body that might be draining your system and preventing you from achieving oral health.

Takeaways

- Some people never get cavities; others get cavities no matter how hard they work on dental health.

- Your oral microbiome is a complex outcome of interrelationships between genetics, microbes, environment, and immune function.

- While you can't change your genetics or your past, you *can* change your environment and your microbes.

APPENDIX

Summary of Human Commensal Oral Microbiota

GENUS (PHYLUM)	I	A	HABITAT 1	HABITAT 2	HABITAT 3	HABITAT 4	BP
Actinomyces (Actinobacteria)		✓			✓		✓
Butyrivibrio (Firmicutes)			✓				
Capnocytophaga (Bacteroidetes)					✓	✓	
Fusobacterium* (Fusobacteria)	✓	✓				✓	
Gemella* (Firmicutes)	✓			✓		✓	
Granulicatella (Firmicutes)	✓						✓
Haemophilus (Proteobacteria)	✓	✓			✓		✓
Leptotrichia (Fusobacteria)	✓				✓		
Neisseria* (Proteobacteria)	✓	✓	✓		✓	✓	
Rothia* (Actinobacteria)	✓	✓	✓		✓		
Streptococcus** (Firmicutes)	✓	✓	✓	✓	✓	✓	
Veillonella* (Firmicutes)	✓	✓	✓			✓	✓

* Dominant genera of the oral cavity

** The most abundant genera of the oral cavity[164]

TABLE KEY

I	Infants
A	Adults
Habitat 1	Saliva, tongue, throat, tonsils
Habitat 2	Cheek, gums, roof of the mouth
Habitat 3	Supragingival dental plaque
Habitat 4	Subgingival dental plaque
BP	Lowers blood pressure

Oral Microbes Involved in Disease

DISEASE	ORAL MICROBES
Cavities	Actinomyces, *S. mitis*, *S. mutans*, *S. salivarius*, *S. sobrinus*, Candida
Infected root canals	*Fusobacterium nucleatum*, *Porphyromonas endodontalis*, *Prevotella baroniae*, *Tannerella forsythia*
Gingivitis	Actinobacillus, Campylobacter, *Fusobacterium nucleatum*, *Porphyromonas gingivalis*
Periodontitis	*Eubacterium saphenum*, *Parvimonas micra*, *Prevotella denticola*, *Prevotella gingivalis*, *Treponema denticola*, *Treponema forsythia*
Atherosclerotic plaques	*Fusobacterium nucleatum*, Neisseria, *Prevotella gingivalis*, *Streptococcus sanguinis*, *Treponema denticola*, *Treponema forsythia*
Rheumatoid arthritis joints	*Prevotella intermedia*, *Fusobacterium nucleatum*, *Serratia proteamaculans*
"Pathogenic bacteria" common in healthy mouths	Bifidobacteriaceae species, *Haemophilus influenza*, *Moraxella catarrhalis*, *Neisseria meningitides*, *Porphyromonas gingivalis*, *Streptococcus pneumoniae*, *Streptococcus pyogenes*, Treponema species

Physician-Dentist Letter

What Physicians Should Consider When Treating Patients With Periodontal Disease

Dear Physician:

Often overlooked when considering CRP is the contribution of gum disease (an infection in the mouth). When you are treating your patient using CRP levels as an indicator of health, or to assess treatment efficacy, it's essential to keep the patient's oral health status, and how it affects CRP, in context with the medical treatment.

For example, if your patient has heart disease, it's likely that the patient's gum disease is contributing to the heart disease. The clinical research now suggests that the correlation between CRP and gum disease might be an underlying mechanism in the association between gum disease and a higher risk for heart disease.

Another potential area of concern is the root canal. Studies show there's **no legitimate connection** between CRP and root canals. However, there **is** a connection between CRP and infection of the teeth. A failed root canal is an infected tooth and should be treated as part of assessing CRP.

Give this letter (beginning on the next page) to your patient's dentist to fill out and return to you to help you make a more complete CRP assessment.

Thank you for taking the time to review this letter and taking a global view of our patients' care.

Some studies for further reading:
http://www.ncbi.nlm.nih.gov/pubmed/11577954
http://www.nutritionandmetabolism.com/content/9/1/88

Mark Burhenne DDS
Mark Burhenne DDS

Physician-Dentist CRP Letter
Created by Mark Burhenne DDS

I grant full permission for this letter to be emailed, shared, and reprinted. While you are under no obligation to do so, I always appreciate a link back to the original at
askthedentist.com/crp-and-oral-health

Dear Dentist:

I am currently seeing our mutual patient, _____, and using CRP as a measure for diagnosis and treatment. I recognize that oral health is a contributor to CRP and thus need to know the status of our patient's oral health.

Select the general state of oral health (could be more than one):

❑ **No gum disease:** Perfect gum health. *Assessment: No contribution to CRP levels.*

❑ **Aggressive periodontitis:** Clinically healthy patients, but have rapid attachment loss and bone destruction and a family history. *Assessment: Likely strong contribution to CRP levels.*

❑ **Chronic periodontitis:** Most frequently occurring form, characterized by inflammation of all the supporting tissues of the teeth and eventual progressive loss of attachment and bone loss and formation of deep pockets. This usually occurs slowly, over a period of time, and can happen in stages. *Assessment: Likely strong contribution to CRP levels.*

❑ **Periodontitis as manifestation of systemic disease:** Typically begins at a young age. Systemic diseases such as heart diseases, respiratory diseases, and diabetes are linked to this form of periodontitis. *Assessment: Likely strong contribution to CRP levels.*

❑ **Necrotizing periodontal disease:** This is an infection characterized by the death of gingival tissues, periodontal ligament, and alveolar bone. These forms of periodontitis are most commonly observed in patients with severe systemic conditions such as HIV, malnutrition, and immune suppression. *Assessment: Likely strong contribution to CRP levels.*

❑ **Failed root canal:** Because infection within the mouth can tax the immune system, root canals should be checked by a cone beam (3D) scan every 2-5 years if possible to check for lesions resulting from failure of the procedure. *Assessment: Likely moderate-to-strong contribution to CRP levels, depending on extent of infection.*

Physician-Dentist CRP Letter
Created by Mark Burhenne DDS

I grant full permission for this letter to be emailed, shared, and reprinted. While you are under no obligation to do so, I always appreciate a link back to the original at
askthedentist.com/crp-and-oral-health

What is the classification of periodontal disease? (ADA AAP Classification of Periodontal Disease)

- ❏ Type I/Gingivitis
- ❏ Type II/Early Periodontitis
- ❏ Type III/Moderate Periodontitis
- ❏ Type IV/Advanced Periodontitis
- ❏ Type V/Refractory & Juvenile Periodontitis

What is the long-term prognosis? When will the inflammatory disease in the mouth be arrested or no longer contribute to CRP?

Have all root canals been assessed by cone beam scan for failure? Please circle Yes or No.

Yes   No

When was the most recent cone beam scan completed on the patient's root canals? Check the box that applies.

- ❏ Less than 2 years
- ❏ 2-5 years
- ❏ 5+ years
- ❏ Never

Physician-Dentist CRP Letter
Created by Mark Burhenne DDS

I grant full permission for this letter to be emailed, shared, and reprinted. While you are under no obligation to do so, I always appreciate a link back to the original at
askthedentist.com/crp-and-oral-health

Page 2/2

NOTES

1. Peter Turnbaugh, Ruth Ley, Micah Hamady, et al., "The Human Microbiome Project: Exploring the Microbial Part of Ourselves in a Changing World," *Nature* 449, no. 7164 (2007): 804–810, doi: 10.1038/nature06244.

2. Jonathan Baker, Batbileg Bor, Melissa Agnello, et al., "Ecology of the Oral Microbiome: Beyond Bacteria," *Trends in Microbiology* 25, no. 5 (2017): 362–374, doi: 10.1016/j.tim.2016.12.012.

3. John Travis, "All the World's a Phage: Viruses That Eat Bacteria Abound—And Surprise," *Science News* 164, no. 2 (2003): 26, https://www.sciencenews.org/article/all-worlds-phage.

4. S. R. Gill, M. Pop, R. T. Deboy, et al., "Metagenomic Analysis of the Human Distal Gut Microbiome," *Science* 312, no. 5778 (2006): 1355–59.

5. Nobuhiko Kamada, Sang-Uk Seo, Grace Chen, et al., "Role of the Gut Microbiota in Immunity and Inflammatory Disease," *Nature Reviews Immunology* 13, no. 5 (2013): 321–335, doi: 10.1038/nri3430.

6. Ariane Panzer AR and Susan Lynch, "Influence and Effect of the Human Microbiome in Allergy and Asthma," *Current Opinion in Rheumatology* 27, no. 4 (2015): 373–380, doi: 10.1097/BOR.0000000000000191.

7. Thomas Abrahamsson, Hedvig Jakobsson, Anders Andersson, et al., "Low Diversity of the Gut Microbiota in Infants with Atopic Eczema," *The Journal of Allergy and Clinical Immunology* 129, no. 2 (2012): 434–440, 440 e431–432, doi: 10.1016/j.jaci.2011.10.025.

8. Kaarina Kukkonen, Erkki Savilahti, Tari Haahtela, et al., "Probiotics and Prebiotic Galacto-Oligosaccharides in the Prevention of Allergic Diseases: A Randomized, Double-Blind, Placebo-Controlled Trial," *The Journal of Allergy and Clinical Immunology* 119, no. 1 (2007): 192–198, doi: 10.1016/j.jaci.2006.09.009.

9. Christina West, "Gut Microbiota and Allergic Disease: New Findings," *Current Opinion in Clinical Nutrition and Metabolic Care* 17, no. 3 (2014): 261–266, doi: 10.1097/MCO.0000000000000044.

10. Mogens Kilian, Iain Chapple, M. Hannig, et al., "The Oral Microbiome— An Update for Oral Healthcare Professionals," *British Dental Journal* 221, no. 10 (2016): 657–666, doi: 10.1038/sj.bdj.2016.865.

11. "History of Dentistry Timeline," American Dentist Association, Accessed Nov 28, 2018, https://www.ada.org/en/about-the-ada/ada-history-and-presidents-of-the-ada/ada-history-of-dentistry-timeline.

12. William Wade, "Unculturable Bacteria—The Uncharacterized Organisms That Cause Oral Infections," *Journal of the Royal Society of Medicine* 95, no. 2 (2002): 81–83, https://www.ncbi.nlm.nih.gov/pmc/articles/PMC1279316.

13. Michael Rappé and Stephen Giovannoni, "The Uncultured Microbial Majority," *Annual Review of Microbiology* 57 (2003): 369–394, doi: 10.1146/annurev.micro.57.030502.090759.

14. Floyd Dewhirst, Tuste Chen, Jacques Izard, et al., "The Human Oral Microbiome," *Journal of Bacteriology* 192, no. 19 (2010): 5002–5017, doi: 10.1128/JB.00542-10.

15. "Microbiology by Numbers," *Nature Reviews Microbiology* 9 (2011): 628, doi: 10.1038/nrmicro2644.

16. Arianna DeGruttola, Daren Low, Atsushi Mizoguchi, et al., "Current Understanding of Dysbiosis in Disease in Human and Animal Models," *Inflammatory Bowel Diseases* 22, no. 5 (2016): 1137–1150, doi: 10.1097/MIB.0000000000000750.

17. Ingegerd Johansson, Ewa Witkowska, B. Kaveh, et al., "The Microbiome in Populations with a Low and High Prevalence of Caries," *Journal of Dental Research* 95, no. 1 (2016): 80–86, doi: 10.1177/0022034515609554.

18. Arianna DeGruttola, et al., "Current Understanding of Dysbiosis in Disease in Human and Animal Models."

19. C. Lee Ventola, "The Antibiotic Resistance Crisis: Part 1: Causes and Threats." *P & T* 40, no. 4 (2015): 277–283, https://www.ncbi.nlm.nih.gov/pubmed/25859123.

20. Catherine Lozupone, Jesse Stombaugh, Jeffrey Gordon, et al., "Diversity, Stability and Resilience of the Human Gut Microbiota," *Nature* 489, no. 7415 (2012): 220–230, doi: 10.1038/nature11550.

21. Les Dethlefsen and David Relman, "Incomplete Recovery and Individualized Responses of the Human Distal Gut Microbiota to Repeated Antibiotic Perturbation," *PNAS* 108 Supplement 1 (2011): 4554–4561, doi: 10.1073/pnas.1000087107.

22. Grave Lee, Kelly Reveles, Russell Attridge, et al., "Outpatient Antibiotic Prescribing in the United States: 2000 to 2010," *BMC Medicine* 12, no. 96 (2014), doi: 10.1186/1741-7015-12-96.

23. G. Vighi, F. Marcucci, L. Sensi, et al., "Allergy and the Gastrointestinal System," *Clinical and Experimental Immunology* 153, Supplement 1 (2008): 3–6, doi: 10.1111/j.1365-2249.2008.03713.x.

24. Deirdre Devine, Philip Marsh, Josephine Meade, "Modulation of Host Responses by Oral Commensal Bacteria," *Journal of Oral Microbiology* 7 (2015), doi: 10.3402/jom.v7.26941.

25. Ensanya Ali Abou Neel, Anas Aljabo, Adam Strange, et al., "Demineralization-Remineralization Dynamics in Teeth and Bone," *International Journal of Nanomedicine* 11 (2016): 4743–4763, doi: 10.2147/ IJN.S107624.

26. Ibid.

27. Ibid.

28. Izabela Struzycka, "The Oral Microbiome in Dental Caries," *Polish Journal of Microbiology / Polskie Towarzystwo Mikrobiologow = The Polish Society of Microbiologists* 63, no. 2 (2014): 127–135, https://www .ncbi.nlm.nih.gov/pubmed/25115106.

29. Jinzhi He, Yan Li, Yangpei Cao, et al., "The Oral Microbiome Diversity and Its Relation to Human Diseases," *Folia Microbiologica* 60, no. 1 (2015): 69–80, doi: 10.1007/s12223-014-0342-2.

30. Jukka Meurman and Iva Stamatova, "Probiotics: Contributions to Oral Health," *Oral Diseases* 13, no. 5 (2007): 443–451, doi: 10.1111/ j.1601-0825.2007.01386.x.

31. Hiroshi Kiyono and Tatsuhiko Azegami, "The Mucosal Immune System: From Dentistry to Vaccine Development," Proceedings of the Japan Academy Series B, Physical and Biological Sciences 91, no. 8 (2015): 423–439, doi: 10.2183/pjab.91.423.

32. Ruiqing Wu, Dunfang Zhang, Eric Tu, et al., "The Mucosal Immune System in the Oral Cavity—An Orchestra of T Cell Diversity," *International Journal of Oral Science* 6, no. 3 (2014): 125–132, doi: 10.1038/ijos.2014.48.

33. Jukka Meurman, et al., "Probiotics: Contributions to Oral Health."

34. Ruiqing Wu, et al., "The Mucosal Immune System in the Oral Cavity—An Orchestra of T Cell Diversity."

35. Koichi Shudo, Hiroshi Fukasawa, Madoka Nakagomi, et al., "Towards Retinoid Therapy For Alzheimer's Disease," *Current Alzheimer Research* 6, no. 3 (2009): 302–311, doi: 10.2174/156720509788486581.

36. Alessio Fasano, "Leaky Gut and Autoimmune Diseases," *Clinical Reviews in Allergy and Immunology* 42, no. 1 (2012): 71–78, doi: 10.1007/ s12016-011-8291-x.

37. Hiroshi Kiyono, et al., "The Mucosal Immune System: From Dentistry to Vaccine Development."

38. Magali Noval Rivas and Talal Chatila, "Regulatory T Cells in Allergic Diseases," *The Journal of Allergy and Clinical Immunology* 138, no. 3 (2016): 639–652, doi: 10.1016/j.jaci.2016.06.003.

39. Deirdre Devine, et al., "Modulation of Host Responses by Oral Commensal Bacteria."

40. Alessio Fasano, "Zonulin, Regulation of Tight Junctions, and Autoimmune Diseases," *Annals of the New York Academy of Sciences* 1258, no. 1 (2012): 25–33, doi: 10.1111/j.1749-6632.2012.06538.x.

41. Alessio Fasano, "Leaky Gut and Autoimmune Diseases," *Clinical Reviews in Allergy and Immunology* 42, no. 1 (2012): 71–78, doi: 10.1007/s12016-011-8291-x.

42. Alessio Fasano and Terez Shea-Donohue, "Mechanisms of Disease: The Role of Intestinal Barrier Function in the Pathogenesis of Gastrointestinal Autoimmune Diseases," *Nature Clinical Practice* 2, no. 9 (2005): 416–422, doi: 10.1038/ncpgasthep0259.

43. Mogens Kilian, et al., "The Oral Microbiome—An Update for Oral Healthcare Professionals."

44. Floyd Dewhirst, et al., "The Human Oral Microbiome."

45. Ibid.

46. I. Cho and M. J. Blaser, "The Human Microbiome: At the Interface of Health and Disease," *Nature Reviews Genetics* 13, no. 4 (2012): 260–70.

47. Y. J. Huang, B. J. Marsland, S. Bunyavanich, et al., "The Microbiome in Allergic Disease," *The Journal of Allergy and Clinical Immunology* 139, no. 4 (2017): 1099–1110.

48. Nicola Segata, Susan Kinder Haake, Peter Mannon, et al., "Composition of the Adult Digestive Tract Bacterial Microbiome Based on Seven Mouth Surfaces, Tonsils, Throat and Stool Samples," *Genome Biology* 13, no. 6 (2012): R42, doi: 10.1186/gb-2012-13-6-r42.

49. Purnima Kumar and Matthew Mason, "Mouthguards: Does the Indigenous Microbiome Play a Role in Maintaining Oral Health?" *Frontiers in Cellular and Infection Microbiology* 6, no. 5 (2015): 35, doi: 10.3389/fcimb.2015.00035.

50. B. Wilson and K. Whelan, "Prebiotic Inulin-Type Fructans and Galacto-Oligosaccharides," *Journal of Gastroenterology and Hepatology* 32, suppl. no. 1 (2017): 64–68.

51. Thomas Auchtung, Tatiana Fofanova, Christopher Stewart, et al., "Investigating Colonization of the Healthy Adult Gastrointestinal Tract by Fungi," *mSphere* 3, no. 2 (2018), doi: 10.1128/mSphere.00092-18.

52. Jinzhi He, et al., "The Oral Microbiome Diversity and Its Relation to Human Diseases."

53. Anna Edlund, Tasha Santiago-Rodriguez, Tobias Boehm, et al., "Bacteriophage and Their Potential Roles in the Human Oral Cavity," *Journal of Oral Microbiology* 7, no. 27423 (2015), doi: 10.3402/jom.v7.27423.

54. Jinzhi He, et al., "The Oral Microbiome Diversity and Its Relation to Human Diseases."

55. Ingegerd Johansson, et al., "The Microbiome in Populations with a Low and High Prevalence of Caries."

56. Elizabeth Thursby and Nathalie Juge, "Introduction to the Human Gut Microbiota," *The Biochemical Journal* 474, no. 11 (2017): 1823–1836, doi: 10.1042/BCJ20160510.

57. P. Lif Holgerson, L. Harnevik, O. Hernell, et al., "Mode of Birth Delivery Affects Oral Microbiota in Infants," *Journal of Dental Research* 90, no. 10 (2011): 1183–1188, doi: 10.1177/0022034511418973.

58. Elizabeth Thursby, et al., "Introduction to the Human Gut Microbiota."

59. P. Lif Holgerson, et al., "Mode of Birth Delivery Affects Oral Microbiota in Infants."

60. Y. J. Huang, et al., "The Microbiome in Allergic Disease."

61. Katherine Gregory, Buck Samuel, Pearl Houghteling, et al., "Influence of Maternal Breast Milk Ingestion on Acquisition of the Intestinal Microbiome in Preterm Infants," *Microbiome* 4, no. 68 (2016): 68, doi: 10.1186/s40168-016-0214-x.

62. Camilia Martin, Pei-Ra Ling, and George Blackburn, "Review of Infant Feeding: Key Features of Breast Milk and Infant Formula," *Nutrients* 8, no. 5 (2016): 279, doi: 10.3390/nu8050279.

63. Rodney Donlan, "Biofilms: Microbial Life on Surfaces," *Emerging Infectious Diseases* 8, no. 9 (2002): 881–890, doi: 10.3201/eid0809.020063.

64. Floyd Dewhirst, et al., "The Human Oral Microbiome."

65. Rodney Donlan, "Biofilms: Microbial Life on Surfaces."

66. Ibid.

67. Melissa Miller and Bonnie Bassler, "Quorum Sensing in Bacteria," *Annual Review of Microbiology* 55 (2001): 165–199, doi: 10.1146/annurev.micro.55.1.165.

68. B. Wilson, et al., "Prebiotic Inulin-Type Fructans and Galacto-Oligosaccharides."

69. Joanne Slavin, "Fiber and Prebiotics: Mechanisms and Health Benefits," *Nutrients* 5, no. 4 (2013): 1417–1435, doi: 10.3390/nu5041417.

70. Floyd Dewhirst, et al., "The Human Oral Microbiome."

71. Ingegerd Johansson, et al., "The Microbiome in Populations with a Low and High Prevalence of Caries."

72. Maria Cagetti, Stefano Mastroberardino, Egle Milia, et al., "The Use of Probiotic Strains in Caries Prevention: A Systematic Review," *Nutrients* 5, no. 7 (2013): 2530–2550, doi: 10.3390/nu5072530.

73. Prodegin: Lactobacillus Support for Oral Health and Weight Management. Reno, NV: Klaire Labs, a division of ProThera;2011.

74. Jinzhi He, et al., "The Oral Microbiome Diversity and Its Relation to Human Diseases."

75. Izabela Struzycka, "The Oral Microbiome in Dental Caries."

76. Ibid.

77. Jinzhi He, et al., "The Oral Microbiome Diversity and Its Relation to Human Diseases."

78. E. A. Grice and J. A. Segre, "The Human Microbiome: Our Second Genome," *Annual Review of Genomics and Human Genetics* 13 (2012): 151–71.

79. Ingegerd Johansson, et al., "The Microbiome in Populations with a Low and High Prevalence of Caries."

80. Ibid.

81. Ensanya Ali Abou Neel, et al., "Demineralization-Remineralization Dynamics in Teeth and Bone."

82. Ingegerd Johansson, et al., "The Microbiome in Populations with a Low and High Prevalence of Caries."

83. Clifton Bingham and Malini Moni, "Periodontal Disease and Rheumatoid Arthritis: The Evidence Accumulates for Complex Pathobiologic Interactions," *Current Opinion in Rheumatology* 25, no. 3 (2013): 345–353, doi: 10.1097/BOR.0b013e32835fb8ec.

84. Karen Schwarzberg, Rosalin Le, Balambal Bharti, et al., "The Personal Human Oral Microbiome Obscures the Effects of Treatment on Periodontal Disease," *PLoS ONE* 9, no. 1 (2014): e86708, doi: 10.1371/journal.pone.0086708.

85. J. Henry Clarke, "Toothaches and Death," *Journal of the History of Dentistry* 47, no. 1 (1999): 11–13, doi: https://ohsu.pure.elsevier.com/en/publications/toothaches-and-death-2.

86. S. Porter and C. Scully, "Oral Malodour (Halitosis)," *BMJ* 333, no. 7569 (2006): 632–635, doi: 10.1136/bmj.38954.631968.AE.

87. Ibid.

88. Walter Loesche, "Microbiology of Dental Decay and Periodontal Disease," in *Medical Microbiology*, 4th ed., edited by Samuel Baron (Galveston, TX: University of Texas Medical Branch at Galveston; 1996).

89. Ingegerd Johansson, et al., "The Microbiome in Populations with a Low and High Prevalence of Caries."

90. Maria Cagetti, et al., "The Use of Probiotic Strains in Caries Prevention: A Systematic Review."

91. Clifton Bingham, et at., "Periodontal Disease and Rheumatoid Arthritis: The Evidence Accumulates for Complex Pathobiologic Interactions."

92. E. A. Grice, et al., "The Human Microbiome: Our Second Genome."

93. Jinzhi He, et al., "The Oral Microbiome Diversity and Its Relation to Human Diseases."

94. Nicola Segata, et al., "Composition of the Adult Digestive Tract Bacterial Microbiome Based on Seven Mouth Surfaces, Tonsils, Throat and Stool Samples."

95. Ibid.

96. Ingegerd Johansson, et al., "The Microbiome in Populations with a Low and High Prevalence of Caries."

97. Michael Docktor, Bruce Paster, Shelly Abramowicz, et al., "Alterations in Diversity of the Oral Microbiome in Pediatric Inflammatory Bowel Disease," *Inflammatory Bowel Diseases* 18, no. 5 (2012): 935–942, doi: 10.1002/ibd.21874.

98. Michael Gershon, "Review Article: Serotonin Receptors and Transporters—Roles in Normal and Abnormal Gastrointestinal Motility," *Alimentary Pharmacology & Therapeutics* 20, Supplement 7 (2004): 3–14, doi: 10.1111/j.1365-2036.2004.02180.x.

99. Jinzhi He, et al., "The Oral Microbiome Diversity and Its Relation to Human Diseases."

100. Hiroshi Kiyono, et al., "The Mucosal Immune System: From Dentistry to Vaccine Development."

101. Nicola Segata, et al., "Composition of the Adult Digestive Tract Bacterial Microbiome Based on Seven Mouth Surfaces, Tonsils, Throat and Stool Samples."

102. Ibid.

103. Izabela Struzycka, "The Oral Microbiome in Dental Caries."

104. Yoshio Yamaoka, "Mechanisms of Disease: Helicobacter Pylori Virulence Factors," *Nature Reviews Gastroenterology & Hepatology* 7, no. 11 (2010): 629–641, doi: 10.1038/nrgastro.2010.154.

105. Marjorie Walker and Nicholas Talley, "Review Article: Bacteria and Pathogenesis of Disease in the Upper Gastrointestinal Tract—Beyond the Era of Helicobacter Pylori," *Alimentary Pharmacology & Therapeutics* 39, no. 8 (2014): 767–779, doi: 10.1111/apt.12666.

106. Aaron Thrift, Nirmala Pandeya, Kylie Smith, et al., "Helicobacter Pylori Infection and the Risks of Barrett's Oesophagus: A Population-Based Case-Control Study," *International Journal of Cancer* 130, no. 10 (2012): 2407–2416, doi: 10.1002/ijc.26242.

107. Pradeep Anand, K. Nandakumar, and Trivikrama Shenoy, "Are Dental Plaque, Poor Oral Hygiene, and Periodontal Disease Associated with Helicobacter Pylori Infection?" *Journal of Periodontology* 20, no. 19 (2006): 692–698, doi: 10.3748/wjg.v20.i19.5639.

108. Chun-Ling Jia, Guang-Shui Jiang, Chun-Hai Li, et al., "Effect of Dental Plaque Control on Infection of Helicobacter Pylori in Gastric Mucosa," *Journal of Periodontology* 80, no. 10 (2012): 1069–1073, doi: 10.1902/jop.2009.090029.

109. Siew Ng, Hai Yun Shi, Nima Hamidi, et al., "Worldwide Incidence and Prevalence of Inflammatory Bowel Disease in the 21st Century: A Systematic Review of Population-Based Studies," *The Lancet* 390, 10114 (2018): 2769–2778.

110. Andrew Yu, Louis Cabanilla, Eric Qiong Wu, et al., "The Costs of Crohn's Disease in the United States and Other Western Countries: A Systematic Review," *Current Medical Research and Opinion* 24, no. 2 (2008): 319–328, doi: 10.1185/030079908X260790.

111. Michael Docktor, et al., "Alterations in Diversity of the Oral Microbiome in Pediatric Inflammatory Bowel Disease."

112. Kewir Nyuyki and Quentin Pittman, "Toward a Better Understanding of the Central Consequences of Intestinal Inflammation," *Annals of the New York Academy of Sciences* 1351, no. 1 (2015): 149–154, doi: 10.1111/nyas.12935.

113. Michael Docktor, et al., "Alterations in Diversity of the Oral Microbiome in Pediatric Inflammatory Bowel Disease."

114. Ibid.

115. Fernanda Brito, Cyrla Zaltman, Ana Teresa Pugas Carvalho, et al., "Subgingival Microflora in Inflammatory Bowel Disease Patients with Untreated Periodontitis," *European Journal of Gastroenterology & Hepatology* 25, no. 2 (2012): 239–45, doi: 10.1097/MEG.0b013e32835a2b70.

116. Stephan Vavricka, Christine Manser, Sebastian Hediger, et al., "Periodontitis and Gingivitis in Inflammatory Bowel Disease: A Case-Control Study," *Inflammatory Bowel Diseases* 19, no. 13 (2013): 2768–2777, doi: 10.1097/01.MIB.0000438356.84263.3b.

117. Clifton Bingham, et at., "Periodontal Disease and Rheumatoid Arthritis: The Evidence Accumulates for Complex Pathobiologic Interactions."

118. Bradley Bale, Amy Doneen, and David Vigerust, "High-Risk Periodontal Pathogens Contribute to the Pathogenesis of Atherosclerosis," *BMJ Postgraduate Medical Journals* 93, no. 1098 (2017): 215–220, https://pmj.bmj.com/content/93/1098/215.

119. Ibid.

120. Stefan Reichert, Axel Schlitt, V. Beschow, et al., "Use of Floss/Interdental Brushes is Associated with Lower Risk for New Cardiovascular Events among Patients with Coronary Heart Disease," *Journal of Periodontal Research* 50, no. 2 (2015): 180–188, doi: 10.1111/jre.12191.

121. Curtis Steyers III and Francis Miller Jr., "Endothelial Dysfunction in Chronic Inflammatory Diseases," *International Journal of Molecular Sciences* 15, no. 7 (2014): 11324–11349, doi: 10.3390/ijms150711324.

122. Bradley Bale, et al., "High-Risk Periodontal Pathogens Contribute to the Pathogenesis of Atherosclerosis."

123. Herbert Cobe, "Transitory Bacteremia," *Oral Surgery, Oral Medicine, and Oral Pathology* 7, no. 6 (1954): 609–615, doi: 10.1016/0030-4220(54)90071-7.

124. Bradley Bale, et al., "High-Risk Periodontal Pathogens Contribute to the Pathogenesis of Atherosclerosis."

125. Jukka Meurman, "Oral Microbiota and Cancer," *Journal of Oral Microbiology* 2 (2010), doi: 10.3402/jom.v2i0.5195.

126. Jinzhi He, et al., "The Oral Microbiome Diversity and Its Relation to Human Diseases."

127. Jukka Meurman, "Oral Microbiota and Cancer."

128. Bradley Bale, et al., "High-Risk Periodontal Pathogens Contribute to the Pathogenesis of Atherosclerosis."

129. Embriette Hyde, Fernando Andrade, Zalman Vaksman, et al., "Metagenomic Analysis of Nitrate-Reducing Bacteria in the Oral Cavity: Implications for Nitric Oxide Homeostasis," *PLoS ONE* 9, no. 3 (2014): e88645, doi: 10.1371/journal.pone.0088645.

130. Jinzhi He, et al., "The Oral Microbiome Diversity and Its Relation to Human Diseases."

131. Clifton Bingham, et at., "Periodontal Disease and Rheumatoid Arthritis: The Evidence Accumulates for Complex Pathobiologic Interactions."

132. Vilana Araujo, Iracema Melo, and Vilma Lima, "Relationship between Periodontitis and Rheumatoid Arthritis: Review of the Literature," *Mediators of Inflammation* 2015 (2015): 259074, doi: 10.1155/2015/259074.

133. Clifton Bingham, et at., "Periodontal Disease and Rheumatoid Arthritis: The Evidence Accumulates for Complex Pathobiologic Interactions."

134. Vilana Araujo, et al., "Relationship between Periodontitis and Rheumatoid Arthritis: Review of the Literature."

135. YiPing Weng Han, Xueyan Wang, "Mobile Microbiome: Oral Bacteria in Extra-Oral Infections and Inflammation," *Journal of Dental Research* 92, no. 6 (2013): 485–491, doi: 10.1177/0022034513487559.

136. Ger Pruijn, Allan Wiik, Walther van Venrooij, "The Use of Citrullinated Peptides and Proteins for the Diagnosis of Rheumatoid Arthritis," *Arthritis Research & Therapy* 12, no. 1 (2010): 203, doi: 10.1186/ar2903.

137. Clifton Bingham, et at., "Periodontal Disease and Rheumatoid Arthritis: The Evidence Accumulates for Complex Pathobiologic Interactions."

138. Vilana Araujo, et al., "Relationship between Periodontitis and Rheumatoid Arthritis: Review of the Literature."

139. Muhammad Nazir, "Prevalence of Periodontal Disease, Its Association with Systemic Diseases and Prevention," *International Journal of Health Sciences* 11, no. 12 (2017): 72–80.

140. Antonio Bascones-Martinez, Paula Matesanz-Perez, Marta Escribano-Bermejo, et al., "Periodontal Disease and Diabetes-Review of the Literature," *Medicina Oral, Patologia Oral Y Cirugia Bucal* 16, no. 6 (2011): e722–729.

141. Ibid.

142. G. Scardina and P. Messina, "Good Oral Health and Diet," *Journal of Biomedicine & Biotechnology* 2012 (2012): 720692, doi: 10.1155/2012/720692.

143. M. G. Dominguez-Bello, K. M. De Jesus-Laboy, N. Shen, et al., "Partial Restoration of the Microbiota of Cesarean-Born Infants Via Vaginal Microbial Transfer," *Nature Magazine* 22, no. 3 (2016): 250–53.

144. Aparna Sheetal, Vinay Kumar Hiremath, Anand Patil, et al., "Malnutrition and Its Oral Outcome—A Review," *Journal of Clinical and Diagnostic Research* 7, no. 1 (2013): 178–180, doi: 10.7860/JCDR/2012/5104.2702.

145. Gian Paolo Littarru, Ryo Nakamura, Lester Ho, et al., "Deficiency of Coenzyme Q 10 in Gingival Tissue from Patients with Periodontal Disease," *Proceedings of the National Academy of Sciences of the United States of America* 68, no. 10 (1971): 2332–2335, http://www.ncbi.nlm.nih.gov/pubmed/5289867.

146. Sathish Manthena, Mulpuri Rao, Lakshmi Penubolu, et al., "Effectiveness of CoQ10 Oral Supplements as an Adjunct to Scaling and Root Planing in Improving Periodontal Health," *Journal of Clinical and Diagnostic Research* 9, no. 8 (2015): Zc26–28, doi: 10.7860/JCDR/2015/13486.6291.

147. Anirban Chatterjee, Abhishek Kandwal, Nidhi Singh, et al., "Evaluation of Co-Q10 Anti-Gingivitis Effect on Plaque Induced Gingivitis: A Randomized Controlled Clinical Trial," *Journal of Indian Society of Periodontology* 16, no. 4 (2012): 539–542, doi: 10.4103/0972-124X.106902.

148. Ingegerd Johansson, et al., "The Microbiome in Populations with a Low and High Prevalence of Caries."

149. Thomas Auchtung, et al., "Investigating Colonization of the Healthy Adult Gastrointestinal Tract by Fungi."

150. Stefan Reichert, et al., "Use of Floss/Interdental Brushes is Associated with Lower Risk for New Cardiovascular Events among Patients with Coronary Heart Disease."

151. D. Belstrom, M. Sembler-Moller, M. Grande, et al. "Impact of Oral Hygiene Discontinuation on Supragingival and Salivary Microbiomes," *JDR Clinical & Translational Research* 3, no. 1 (2017): 57–64, doi: 10.1177/2380084417723625.

152. M. Bashash, M. Marchand, H. Hu, et al., "Prenatal Fluoride Exposure and Thyroid Function Among Adults Living in Canada," *Environmental International* 121 (2018): 658–66.

153. A. J. Malin and C. Till, "Exposure to Fluoridated Water and Attention Deficit Hyperactivity Disorder Symptoms in Children at 6 to 12 Years of Age in Mexico City," *Environmental Health* 14 (2015): 17.

154. M. A. Ciorba, "Gastroenterologist's Guide to Probiotics," *Clinical Gastroenterology and Hepatology* 10, no. 9 (2012): 960–68.

155. M. Seminario-Amez, J. Lopez-Lopez, A. Estrugo-Devesa, et al., "Probiotics and Oral Health: A Systematic Review," *Medicina Oral, Patologia Oral y Cirugia Bucal* 22, no. 3 (2017):e282–e288.

156. Jukka Meurman, et al., "Probiotics: Contributions to Oral Health."

157. M. Seminario-Amez, et al., "Probiotics and Oral Health: A Systematic Review."

158. L. Bonifait, F. Chandad, and D. Grenier, "Probiotics for Oral Health: Myth or Reality?" *Journal of the Canadian Dental Association* 75, no. 8 (2009): 585–90.

159. S. Srinivasan, B. Nandlal, and S. Rao, "Assessment of Plaque Regrowth with a Probiotic Toothpaste Containing Lactobacillus Paracasei: A Spectrophotometric Study," *Journal of the Indian Society of Pedodontics and Preventive Dentistry* 35, no. 4 (2017): 307–311, doi: 10.4103/JISPPD .JISPPD_323_16.

160. Embriette Hyde, et al., "Metagenomic Analysis of Nitrate-Reducing Bacteria in the Oral Cavity: Implications for Nitric Oxide Homeostasis."

161. Alessio Fasano, Anna Sapone, Victor Zevallos, et al., "Nonceliac Gluten Sensitivity," *Gastroenterology* 148, no. 6 (2015): 1195–1204, doi: 10.1053/ j.gastro.2014.12.049.

162. R. S. Lord, J. A. Bralley, eds. *Laboratory Evaluation for Integrative and Functional Medicine.* 2nd edition. Duluth, GA: Metametrix Institute, 2008.

163. Ingegerd Johansson, et al., "The Microbiome in Populations with a Low and High Prevalence of Caries."

164. E. A. Grice, et al., "The Human Microbiome: Our Second Genome."

INDEX

Integrative dentists, 144

Intestinal microbiome. *See* Gut
 microbiome

Intestinal permeability. *See*
 Leaky gut

Kilian, Mogens (et al.), quoted,
 51

Lactobacillus bacteria, 44, 57,
 62–63, 71, 72, 132–33, 141

Lactoferrin, in saliva, 35

Lactoperoxidase, in saliva, 35

Lamina propria, 29–30

Leaky gut, 47, 143

Leaky mouth, 48, 102–103

Lin, Steven, 119

Linnaeus, Carl, and taxonomic
 classification, 61

Lipopolysaccharide (LPS),
 79–80

Lymphatic system, 38, 39

Lymphocytes, 39, 42. *See also*
 ß cells; T cells

Lysozyme, in saliva, 34

M cells, 42

MALT (mucosa-associated
 lymphoid tissue), 38–39, 41, 42

Marshall, Barry, 92

Mercury fillings, 140

Metametrix Clinical Laboratory,
 2, 94, 96

Microbial balance, 22–23;
 131–37; testing, 145–47

Microbial dysbiosis. *See*
 Dysbiosis

Microbiomes, in general, 4–11;
 benefits, 54–55; and dysbiosis,
 20–22; illustrated, 7; microbial
 balance, 22–23, 131–37;
 rainforest analogy, 9–10, 20,
 34, 69; origin, 57–58. *See also*
 specific microbiomes

Microbiota, defined, 5. *See also*
 Good bugs/bad bugs

Microecology, of the mouth,
 72–73

Minerals, 125, 141

Morgan, Heather, quoted, 119

Mouth, 26–36; anatomy,
 illustrated, 29; locations,
 27–28, 38, 90–91; mucosal
 barrier, 28, 29–31, 39–40;
 teeth, 29, 30–33

Mouth-breathing, 130

Mouth tissue, healing, 138–40

Mouthwash, 106, 136–37

Mucin, 30, 40

Mucosa-associated lymphoid
 tissue (MALT), 38–39, 41, 42

Mucosal barrier, 48–49

Mucous membranes, in mouth,
 27–28, 29–31, 36, 39–40

Nash, Ogden, quoted, 81

Naso-pharynx associated
lymphoid tissue (NALT), 39
Neisseria bacteria, 64
Niche, defined, 8, 10, 33–34;
illustrated, 65
Nitric oxide, 106
Nutrition, and oral microbiome,
122–26
Nutritional supplements, 139,
142

Olmstead, Stephen, 97
Omega-3 fatty acids, and
inflammation, 138
Oral DNA labs, 145
Oral dysbiosis, 21
Oral microbiome, 8, 11–12,
51–67, 157; bacterial
composition, illustrated, 7, 65;
and disease, 76, 99–116, 158;
and gut, 41–43, 80–81, 99–116;
interacting forces, 152–55;
origins, 57–58; uniqueness,
56–57. See also Dysbiosis;
Immune system
"The Oral Microbiome—An
Update for Oral Healthcare
Professionals," quoted, 5
Oral microbes, 158
Oral mucosa (epithelial lining),
28, 29–31, 36, 39–40
Oral mycobiome (fungal
microbiome), 56

Oral-systemic connection,
80–81, 99–116
Oral virome, 56
Osteoblasts, 32
Osteoclasts, 32
Otis, Carré, quoted, 17

Parker, Dorothy, quoted, 26
"Pathogenic bacteria," 158
Pathogens, defined, 18; and heart
disease, 103–105. See also
Good bugs/bad bugs
Peptides, citrullinated, 108
Periodontal disease, 45–46,
75–78, 178; illustrated, 77; and
oral probiotics, 132–34; and
other diseases, 76, 100–16;
word origin, 77
Periodontal pockets, illustrated,
76
Periodontitis. See Periodontal
disease
pH, in mouth, 34
Phylum, and classification, 62,
63–66
Physician-dentist letter, 105,
109, 147, 159–61
Plaque, 33, 59–60, 71
Porphyromonas gingivalis (P.
gingivalis), 82, 83, 108
Prebiotics, 61, 119
Pregnancy, 121. See also
Childbirth

Probiotics, 58, 77–78, 80, 131–34, 124, 141; dosage, 131; and pregnancy, 121

Processed foods, 122

Proteins, in saliva, 35

Proteobacteria, 7, 63, 65, 66

Pulp, of tooth, 32; illustrated, 30

Pulp-dentine complex, 31, 32

Pulpectomy, 73. *See also* Root canals

Quantitative polymerase chain reaction (qPCR), 14

Quorum sensing, of biofilm, 60

Rainforest analogy, 9–10, 20, 34, 69

Red complex, 82

Regulatory T cells, 43, 44

Resveratrol, and inflammation, 138

Revitin prebiotic toothpaste, 126

Rheumatoid arthritis (RA), 107–109, 110, 158

Rothia bacteria, 64

Root canals, 71, 73, 81, 158; illustrated 31, 69

Ruiz, Donna, 73–74

Saliva, 34–35, 43, 78, 130; production, 35

Salmonella, 19, 20, 21

Secretory IgA (sIgA), 43, 90, 141; and breastfeeding, 58–59

Serotonin, 87

Short-chain fatty acids, 55; and prebiotics, 61

sIgA. *See* Secretory IgA

Skin microbiome, 7, 8

Smoking, 129–30

Stomach microbiome. *See* Gut microbiome

Stratified, squamous (scaly) epithelial tissue, 30

Streptococcus bacteria, 44, 64, 65, 69, 71, 72, 73, 83, 106–107

Stress, 141–42

Sugar, 72, 73, 75, 77, 122–24

T cells, 42–43, 44

Tannerella forsythia, 82

Taxonomic classification charts, 62, 63

Teeth, 29, 30–33; illustrated, 31, 69, 77

"Terrain," 72–73

Tests and testing, 105, 144–48

Toll-like receptors, 40

Tongue brushing, 78

Tooth brushing, 127, 128

Tooth cavities. *See* Cavities

Tooth enamel, 31; illustrated, 30

Toothpaste, 136; probiotic, 74, 134

Treg cells, 43, 44
Treponema denticola, 82

Urinary tract microbiome, 8

Vaginal childbirth, 120
Vaginal microbiome, 7, 8; and
  childbirth, 57–58, 120
Vaginal seeding, 120–21
Varicella zoster virus, 56
Veillonella bacteria, 64, 106
Viruses, 56; in microbiome, 6–7
Vitamin K, 55
Vitamins, 55, 125–26, 141

Warren, Robin, 92
Water fluoridation, 32, 128–29
Water intake, 130
Waterpik water flosser, 128
Watterson, Bill, quoted, 150
Weight issues, 114
Wheat products, and healing,
  139–40

Yeast. *See* Candida
Yogurt, 124

Zinc carnosine, and healing, 139

ACKNOWLEDGMENTS

I want to thank all of the great writers in my family, both those that were published and those that had a natural gift that was shared only in private communications: Gordon Nelson, Lynn Nelson, Suzannah Davis, Julie Nelson, Anna Dooley, and Mike Dooley. I want to thank my mentors and teachers along the way, of whom there were many: David Puett, Elois Ann Berlin, Brent Berlin, Luz Graciella Joly, Diane Hartle, Clifton Baile, Andy Bralley, and Richard Lord. Thanks to Stephen Olmstead and Klaire Labs, who started me on this fascinating journey. I am grateful to my stellar dental health team, Dr. Ken Hutchinson and dental hygienist Vickie Schwartz, who helped tremendously in my research. Thanks to my beautiful daughter, Aubrey, who put up with my absences while I wrote. And thanks to the love of my life, Jay Prescott, who supported my decision to write this book and helped make it possible in all of the little ways.

ABOUT THE AUTHOR

Cass Nelson-Dooley, MS, studied medicinal plants in the rainforests of Panama in 2003 as a Fulbright Scholar, and then launched a career in science and natural medicine. She researched the pharmacology of medicinal plants at the University of Georgia and AptoTec, Inc., and then joined the innovators at Metametrix Clinical Laboratory and Genova Diagnostics. She enjoys teaching, presenting, writing, and researching how to address the underlying causes of disease, not just the symptoms. She has over a decade of experience teaching doctors about integrative and functional laboratory results. She is the CEO of Health First Consulting, LLC, a medical communications company with the mission to improve human health using the written word. Ms. Nelson-Dooley has published case studies, book chapters, and journal articles about natural medicine, nutrition, laboratory testing, obesity, and osteoporosis.